The DMDD Family Handbook

A Comprehensive Guide to Supporting Your Explosive Child, Protecting Siblings, and Saving Your Marriage from Disruptive Mood Dysregulation Disorder

Cornelia Louise Whitaker

ISBN: 978-1-7643522-4-6

First Edition: 2025

This book is designed to provide helpful information on the subjects discussed. It is not intended as a substitute for professional medical advice, diagnosis, or treatment. Always seek the advice of your physician, psychiatrist, psychologist, or other qualified health provider with any questions you may have regarding a medical or mental health condition. Never disregard professional medical advice or delay in seeking it because of something you have read in this book.

The information provided in this book is based on the author's research, professional experience, and available evidence at the time of publication. Medical and psychological research continuously evolves, and treatment recommendations may change. Readers should consult with qualified healthcare professionals before implementing any treatment strategies or making medical decisions.

The names and scenarios depicted in this book are purely for illustrative purposes only. Any resemblance to actual persons, living or dead, or actual events is purely coincidental. Case examples are composites drawn from clinical experience and research, with identifying details changed to protect privacy and confidentiality. No case example represents any specific individual or family.

This handbook is intended for educational and informational purposes. It does not establish a therapist-client, doctor-patient, or professional relationship between the author and readers. The strategies and recommendations provided should be adapted to individual circumstances in consultation with qualified professionals familiar with your specific situation.

Table of Contents

Chapter 1: What is DMDD?

The phone call from your child's school comes on a Tuesday afternoon. Your seven-year-old threw a desk. Again. The principal uses words like "unacceptable behavior" and "consequences," but you hear something else underneath—bewilderment. They don't understand your child any more than you do. You've tried everything. Time-outs don't work. Rewards barely register. The pediatrician suggested "more structure" as if you haven't color-coded every routine in your household. Then a psychiatrist mentions three letters that change everything: DMDD.

Disruptive Mood Dysregulation Disorder represents one of the newest additions to our understanding of childhood mental health conditions. Added to the Diagnostic and Statistical Manual of Mental Disorders (DSM-5) in 2013, this diagnosis emerged from decades of clinical observation and research showing that certain children experienced chronic irritability and explosive outbursts that didn't fit neatly into existing diagnostic categories. These weren't children having occasional bad days or testing boundaries during developmental phases. These were children whose nervous systems seemed perpetually primed for explosion, whose baseline mood hovered somewhere between irritable and enraged, whose families walked on eggshells wondering which interaction might trigger the next eruption.

The Diagnosis That Changed Everything

DMDD describes a pattern of behavior and mood that extends far beyond typical childhood tantrums or adolescent moodiness. The disorder centers on two core features that must persist for at least twelve consecutive months. First, children with DMDD display severe temper outbursts—verbal rages or physical aggression—that occur on average three or more times per week. These aren't minor upsets. A child with DMDD might scream for thirty minutes because dinner appeared five minutes late, or destroy their bedroom because a sibling looked at them "wrong." Second, between these explosive episodes, the child maintains an irritable or angry mood most of the day, nearly every day. Parents describe their children as having a "short fuse" or being "always on edge."

The diagnosis applies to children between ages six and eighteen, though symptoms typically emerge before age ten. Clinicians won't diagnose DMDD in children younger than six because temper tantrums remain developmentally normal in preschoolers. The condition also requires that symptoms appear in at least two settings—home, school, or with peers—and cause significant impairment in the child's functioning.

Case Example: Marcus, Age 8

Marcus's mother, Jennifer, spent three years watching her son spiral before receiving the DMDD diagnosis. "I thought I was failing as a parent," she recalls. Marcus's day started badly from the moment he woke up. If his socks felt "wrong," he'd throw them across the room and refuse to get dressed, screaming that his mother "ruined everything." The bus ride to school became impossible after Marcus punched another child who accidentally bumped his backpack. Teachers reported that Marcus seemed angry most of the time, snapping at classmates over minor infractions and refusing to transition between activities without loud protests.

The breaking point came during a family dinner. Marcus's younger sister asked to pass the salt, and Marcus erupted. He swept his plate onto the floor, overturned his chair, and screamed that everyone hated him. The outburst lasted forty-five minutes.

Afterward, Marcus seemed genuinely confused about what had happened, asking his mother why she looked so upset. This pattern—explosive rage followed by confusion or remorse—repeated three to five times weekly. Jennifer tried stricter rules, gentler parenting, removing sugar from his diet, and adding more exercise. Nothing changed Marcus's baseline irritability or prevented the explosions.

How DMDD Differs from Other Conditions

Understanding DMDD requires distinguishing it from several other childhood disorders that share overlapping features. This matters because treatment approaches differ significantly based on accurate diagnosis.

Bipolar Disorder was historically the catch-all diagnosis for children showing extreme mood swings and irritability. However, bipolar disorder involves distinct episodes of mania or hypomania—periods of abnormally elevated mood, increased energy, decreased need for sleep, and grandiose thinking. These episodes last for days to weeks, with clear beginnings and endings. Children with DMDD don't experience true manic episodes. Their irritability is chronic and persistent rather than episodic. The child with bipolar disorder might have a week of sleeping three hours nightly while making elaborate plans to start five different businesses, followed by a crash into depression. The child with DMDD wakes up irritable most mornings and stays that way most days, with explosive outbursts punctuating the chronic irritability.

Oppositional Defiant Disorder (ODD) also involves temper outbursts and irritable mood, but children with ODD direct their defiance specifically toward authority figures. The child with ODD might refuse to do homework to spite a teacher or deliberately ignore parental requests. The behavior serves a purpose—to oppose and defy. Children with DMDD don't limit their outbursts to authority figures, and their explosions often

3

seem disconnected from any goal. They might rage at a peer, a sibling, or even themselves with equal intensity.

Autism Spectrum Disorder can include intense tantrums, particularly in response to sensory overload or changes in routine. However, children with autism typically have difficulties with social communication, restricted interests, and sensory sensitivities that explain their outbursts. The child with autism melts down in a crowded, noisy restaurant because the sensory input overwhelms their nervous system. Once removed from the triggering environment, they often regulate. The child with DMDD might explode in any setting, triggered by frustrations that seem minor to observers, and they struggle to regulate even after the trigger disappears.

Attention-Deficit/Hyperactivity Disorder (ADHD) commonly occurs alongside DMDD, making diagnosis more complex. Children with ADHD show impulsivity and difficulty regulating attention, which can lead to frustration and occasional outbursts. But ADHD alone doesn't explain the chronic, severe irritability and frequent explosive episodes characteristic of DMDD. Many children carry both diagnoses.

Case Example: Tanya, Age 10

Tanya's diagnostic journey illustrates these distinctions. Initially diagnosed with bipolar disorder at age seven, Tanya took mood stabilizers for eighteen months with minimal improvement. Her psychiatrist noted that Tanya never showed classic manic symptoms—no decreased sleep paired with increased energy, no pressured speech, no grandiose beliefs. Instead, Tanya seemed perpetually grumpy. She'd wake up cranky, snap at her parents during breakfast, complain about everything at school, and end the day in tears or rage over homework.

Three to four times weekly, something pushed Tanya over the edge. A classmate might make an innocent comment about her haircut, and Tanya would shove the child and storm out of class. At home, running out of her favorite cereal could trigger a thirty-minute tantrum involving thrown objects and accusations that her parents didn't care about her. Between these explosions, Tanya maintained an irritable baseline. She wasn't defying authority specifically—she lashed out at siblings, peers, and adults equally. She wasn't responding to sensory overload—the triggers seemed almost random. She did have ADHD, but stimulant medication improved her attention without touching the irritability or outbursts.

After re-evaluation, Tanya received the DMDD diagnosis. Her mother felt relief mixed with frustration. "Finally, someone named what we'd been living with," she said. "But then I realized how little anyone knew about treating it."

The Neuroscience Behind the Explosions

Understanding the brain mechanisms underlying DMDD helps parents make sense of behavior that seems irrational or manipulative. These children aren't choosing to explode. Their nervous systems process frustration, disappointment, and emotional stimuli differently than typically developing children.

Research using functional magnetic resonance imaging (fMRI) shows that children with DMDD demonstrate altered activity in brain regions responsible for emotion regulation. The amygdala, which processes emotional information and threat detection, shows heightened reactivity to negative facial expressions and frustrating situations. Children with DMDD perceive neutral faces as angry or threatening more often than other children. They misinterpret social cues, seeing hostility where none exists.

The prefrontal cortex, which provides top-down regulation of emotional responses, shows reduced activity during frustrating tasks in children with DMDD. Think of the amygdala as the brain's smoke detector, constantly scanning for danger or frustration. In DMDD, that smoke detector activates too easily, sounding alarms for minor irritations that other children would barely notice. Meanwhile, the prefrontal cortex—the brain's fire department, responsible for calming false alarms—responds sluggishly or ineffectively. The child experiences intense emotional arousal without adequate internal resources to modulate that arousal.

Additional research points to differences in how children with DMDD process rewards and frustration. When faced with frustrating tasks or losing games, children with DMDD show exaggerated physiological stress responses and difficulty disengaging from negative emotions. Their nervous systems shift into fight-or-flight mode more readily and stay there longer. This explains why a minor setback—losing a board game, receiving constructive criticism—can trigger a response that seems wildly disproportionate to the situation.

Neurotransmitter systems likely play roles as well, though research continues. Serotonin, which helps regulate mood and impulse control, and dopamine, involved in reward processing and motivation, both appear implicated in mood dysregulation disorders. This neurobiological foundation explains why behavioral interventions alone often prove insufficient and why medication can help some children.

Case Example: David, Age 9

David's parents struggled to understand his explosive behavior until his psychiatrist explained the neuroscience. David would come home from school seeming fine, then erupt over homework. His parents couldn't figure out what they were doing wrong. The psychiatrist explained that David spent all day at school working intensely to regulate his emotions and hold himself together. His amygdala fired repeatedly as classmates bumped into him in hallways, as teachers gave instructions he found confusing, as the cafeteria noise overwhelmed his senses.

His prefrontal cortex worked overtime trying to suppress his irritability and control his responses.

By the time David arrived home—his safe place—he'd exhausted his regulatory capacity. The homework request became the final straw, not because homework was uniquely terrible, but because David had no regulation left. His brain, already operating in chronic stress mode, couldn't handle one more demand. This framework helped David's parents stop taking the explosions personally and start implementing environmental modifications. They built in decompression time after school before homework. They reduced demands during David's most dysregulated times. They recognized that David's brain needed help doing what came naturally to other children.

Current Research and What We Know (and Don't Know)

DMDD research remains in relatively early stages given the diagnosis's recent introduction. Several areas show active investigation with preliminary but important findings.

Prevalence and Demographics: Studies suggest DMDD affects approximately 2 to 5 percent of children in the general population, with rates higher in clinical settings. The condition appears slightly more common in males than females in community samples, though clinical samples show more balanced gender ratios. DMDD occurs across all socioeconomic and cultural backgrounds.

Course and Outcomes: Longitudinal research provides both concerning and hopeful findings. Children with DMDD show increased risk for developing anxiety disorders and major depression in adolescence and young adulthood. The chronic irritability doesn't typically persist as DMDD into adulthood— the diagnosis officially applies only to those under eighteen— but evolves into other mood and anxiety conditions. Follow-up studies show that young adults with childhood DMDD histories have elevated rates of mood disorders, greater functional impairment, poorer educational outcomes, and more health problems than peers without psychiatric histories. However, early intervention and appropriate treatment significantly improve these trajectories.

Comorbidity Patterns: DMDD rarely occurs alone. Studies show that 63 to 92 percent of children meeting DMDD criteria also meet criteria for at least one other psychiatric disorder. ADHD, anxiety disorders, and ODD frequently co-occur with DMDD, complicating both diagnosis and treatment. This high comorbidity rate raises questions about DMDD's status as a distinct disorder versus a severe presentation of overlapping conditions. Researchers continue examining these relationships.

Treatment Research: Because DMDD is newly recognized, few treatment studies focus specifically on this diagnosis. Most current treatments adapt approaches developed for other childhood disorders associated with irritability, particularly ADHD, ODD, and anxiety disorders. Cognitive-behavioral therapy (CBT) shows promise in helping children identify distorted thinking patterns and develop coping skills. Dialectical behavior therapy adapted for children (DBT-C) teaches emotion regulation skills. Parent training programs help caregivers respond effectively to irritability and prevent escalation. Medication research remains limited, though stimulants, antidepressants, and certain mood stabilizers show potential benefits for some children.

The Matthews Protocol, developed by Dr. Dan Matthews, represents one emerging treatment approach specifically targeting DMDD. This protocol uses a combination of amantadine and oxcarbazepine (Trileptal)—medications with different primary indications—to address the neurological underpinnings of explosive irritability. Preliminary reports suggest success rates above 75 percent in reducing outbursts and irritability, though large-scale controlled trials have not yet been published. The protocol reflects growing recognition that DMDD may respond to treatments targeting specific neurotransmitter systems and neural circuits.

What We Don't Know: Major gaps persist in our understanding. The exact causes of DMDD remain unclear, though research points to interactions between genetic vulnerability, brain development, environmental stress, and early life experiences. We don't yet have validated diagnostic tools or biomarkers—diagnosis relies entirely on clinical observation and parent report. We can't predict which children will respond to which treatments, forcing families through trial-and-error processes. We don't fully understand the relationship between DMDD and other disorders or why some children develop DMDD while others with similar risk factors don't. Long-term outcome research needs expansion, particularly regarding factors that promote resilience and recovery.

These knowledge gaps frustrate families seeking answers and certainty. Living with DMDD means accepting significant uncertainty about causes, optimal treatments, and long-term prognosis. But it also means that each year brings new research, refined understanding, and improved interventions. The diagnosis that changed everything continues changing as our knowledge expands.

Moving Forward from Diagnosis

Receiving a DMDD diagnosis marks both an ending and a beginning. The endless cycle of trying strategies that don't work, hearing that you just need to be stricter or gentler or more consistent, wondering if you're somehow causing your child's difficulties—those doubts can finally rest. The diagnosis provides a framework for understanding behavior that seemed inexplicable. It validates your experience that your child's difficulties exceed normal developmental challenges.

But diagnosis also begins a new journey through treatment options, school accommodations, medication decisions, and daily management strategies. The following chapters address each step of that journey, providing research-based information and practical guidance drawn from both clinical literature and the lived experiences of families who've walked this path before you.

Key Points to Remember

- DMDD involves chronic irritability punctuated by frequent severe outbursts, persisting for at least twelve months across multiple settings

- The disorder differs from bipolar disorder (no manic episodes), ODD (not limited to defiance of authority), and autism (not primarily sensory-based)

- Neurobiological research shows altered functioning in brain regions controlling emotion regulation, with overactive threat detection and underactive emotional control

- DMDD affects 2-5% of children, frequently co-occurs with other conditions, and increases risk for later mood and anxiety disorders

- Research remains limited but growing, with several treatment approaches showing promise though no definitive standard treatment exists yet

- Accurate diagnosis provides essential foundation for accessing appropriate interventions and support systems

Chapter 2: The Diagnostic Journey

You've read the description of DMDD and recognized your child in every sentence. The chronic irritability, the explosive outbursts over seemingly nothing, the constant walking on eggshells—it all fits. But recognition doesn't equal diagnosis. Getting from "I think my child has DMDD" to "My child has been formally diagnosed with DMDD" involves navigating a healthcare system that often knows less about this condition than parents who've spent hours researching online. The diagnostic journey tests patience, persistence, and your capacity to advocate effectively while emotionally depleted.

Recognizing the Signs

Parents usually recognize something isn't right long before receiving a diagnosis. You might notice in your toddler years that tantrums extend well past age four, or that your child's emotional responses seem dramatically more intense than their peers. Maybe kindergarten teachers start commenting on your child's "difficulty with transitions" or "trouble regulating emotions"—code phrases that signal concern without naming the problem directly.

Certain patterns distinguish DMDD from typical childhood behavior challenges. Normal children have tantrums. Children with DMDD have prolonged, intense rages that exhaust everyone involved. Normal children get grumpy sometimes. Children with DMDD maintain an irritable baseline mood most days. Normal children have bad days. Children with DMDD have bad weeks punctuated by terrible days.

The key diagnostic features include:

Severe temper outbursts that involve verbal rage (screaming, threatening, swearing) or physical aggression (hitting, kicking, throwing objects, destroying property). These outbursts seem grossly disproportionate to the triggering situation. A child explodes for thirty minutes because their sandwich was cut into triangles instead of rectangles. They rage at a sibling who accidentally touched their toy. They destroy homework after making a small error.

Frequency matters. Outbursts must average three or more times per week. Some children have daily explosions. Others might have several clustered together followed by a few calmer days, but the average exceeds three weekly.

Chronic irritability between outbursts distinguishes DMDD from conditions involving episodic mood changes. The child seems angry, cranky, or easily annoyed most of the time. Parents describe feeling like their child wakes up on the wrong side of the bed every morning. Teachers note the child seems perpetually dissatisfied or grumpy. Peers learn to avoid the child because interactions so often end badly.

Duration requirements specify that symptoms must persist for twelve or more consecutive months, with no period of three or more months without symptoms. This duration requirement helps distinguish DMDD from temporary behavioral responses to stress, trauma, or life changes.

Multiple settings must show impairment. The behavior can't be limited to home—it must also appear at school, with peers, or in other environments. Some children show more explosions at home because they feel safest dropping their guard there, but the underlying irritability shows up everywhere.

Age considerations place the disorder between ages six and eighteen, with symptom onset before age ten. Healthcare providers won't diagnose DMDD in preschoolers because tantrum behavior remains developmentally expected, or in adults because the clinical presentation changes significantly after adolescence.

Case Example: Emma, Age 7

Emma's parents, Sarah and Tom, spent two years questioning if Emma's behavior fell within normal limits before seeking evaluation. Emma's tantrums started before age two and never stopped. While other children outgrew that phase by age four or five, Emma's rages continued and intensified. By first grade, Emma was exploding multiple times daily at home and several times weekly at school.

Sarah kept a behavior log for one month at her pediatrician's suggestion. The log revealed Emma had severe tantrums averaging five times weekly, lasting fifteen to forty-five minutes each. Triggers included being told no, transitions between activities, schoolwork that felt challenging, perceived unfairness, sensory irritations (tags in clothes, certain food textures), and sometimes no identifiable trigger at all. Between tantrums, Emma maintained what Sarah called a "three out of ten mood"— never genuinely happy, always somewhat grumpy, quick to complain, and prone to negative interpretations of neutral situations.

The behavior log also showed patterns. Weekends with unstructured time saw more explosions. After-school time proved particularly volatile. Minor frustrations triggered major meltdowns. Sarah wrote: "Emma spent twenty minutes screaming that I 'ruined her life' because I bought the wrong brand of yogurt. She threw the yogurt container at me, kicked the refrigerator door repeatedly, and refused to calm down even after I offered to go buy the preferred brand immediately."

This kind of documentation proves crucial during the diagnostic process. Memory fails under stress, and parents often minimize or forget the severity and frequency of episodes. Written records provide objective data that helps clinicians distinguish DMDD from other conditions.

Finding the Right Professionals

Identifying qualified professionals to evaluate and treat DMDD presents challenges. The diagnosis is relatively new, meaning many healthcare providers received their training before DMDD existed as a recognized disorder. Additionally, child mental health specialists remain in short supply in many communities, with wait lists extending months or longer.

Start with your child's pediatrician or family doctor. While primary care physicians typically don't diagnose complex psychiatric conditions, they can provide referrals, rule out medical conditions that might mimic mood dysregulation (thyroid problems, sleep disorders, certain nutritional deficiencies), and document symptoms for specialists. Some pediatricians have training in developmental and behavioral pediatrics and may provide initial screening.

Child psychiatrists specialize in diagnosing and treating mental health conditions in children and adolescents. They complete medical school followed by residency training in psychiatry with specialization in pediatric populations. Psychiatrists can prescribe medications and provide psychotherapy, though many focus primarily on medication management. Finding a child psychiatrist familiar with DMDD specifically may require contacting multiple practices and directly asking about their experience with the disorder.

Child psychologists hold doctoral degrees (PhD or PsyD) in psychology with specialized training in child development and mental health. Psychologists conduct comprehensive psychological evaluations, provide therapy, and develop treatment plans but cannot prescribe medication. Many children benefit from working with both a psychiatrist (for medication management) and a psychologist (for therapy).

Licensed clinical social workers (LCSWs) and licensed professional counselors (LPCs) also provide therapy services and may have expertise in childhood behavioral disorders. While they don't typically conduct formal diagnostic evaluations, they can be invaluable treatment team members providing weekly therapy while a psychiatrist manages medications and monitors diagnosis.

Neuropsychologists conduct detailed assessments examining cognitive functioning, attention, memory, executive function, and emotional regulation. A neuropsychological evaluation can help identify co-occurring conditions like ADHD or learning disabilities and provide detailed information about a child's cognitive profile to guide treatment planning.

Case Example: Michael, Age 9

Michael's parents, Lisa and James, faced a six-month wait for an appointment with a child psychiatrist after their pediatrician suggested evaluation for possible DMDD. During the wait, they worked with their pediatrician to document Michael's symptoms systematically. The pediatrician ordered blood work to rule out anemia, thyroid dysfunction, and vitamin deficiencies. All results came back normal.

Lisa also contacted their school district's special education department, requesting an evaluation under the Individuals with Disabilities Education Act (IDEA). The school conducted assessments and identified that Michael's behavior was significantly impacting his educational performance. The school psychologist couldn't diagnose DMDD—that requires a medical professional—but documented the behavioral patterns consistent with a mood disorder and recommended accommodations pending formal diagnosis.

When the psychiatrist appointment finally arrived, Lisa brought a thick folder including:

- Six months of behavior tracking logs

- Report cards showing declining academic performance and behavioral concerns

- Written statements from three different teachers describing classroom incidents

- The school's evaluation results

- Medical records from the pediatrician

- A written timeline of symptom development from infancy through present

The psychiatrist spent ninety minutes interviewing Lisa and James separately, then met with Michael for thirty minutes. She reviewed all documentation, asked detailed questions about family psychiatric history, and carefully assessed for other potential diagnoses. At the end, she provided a provisional diagnosis of DMDD with co-occurring ADHD, explained her reasoning, and outlined treatment recommendations. Lisa and James felt the extensive preparation made the difference between a rushed, superficial evaluation and a thorough assessment leading to accurate diagnosis.

Common Misdiagnoses and Why They Happen

DMDD's relative newness and symptom overlap with other conditions mean misdiagnosis occurs frequently. Understanding common diagnostic errors helps families recognize when a second opinion might be warranted.

Bipolar disorder was the most common misdiagnosis before DMDD's introduction. Children with chronic irritability and explosive rages were often labeled bipolar, despite not showing true manic episodes. The confusion stems from an earlier, broader interpretation of pediatric bipolar disorder that included chronic irritability as a possible presentation. This misdiagnosis matters because bipolar disorder treatment typically involves mood stabilizers or atypical antipsychotics as first-line medications, which may not be optimal for DMDD and carry significant side effect risks.

Oppositional defiant disorder shares features with DMDD, including temper outbursts and irritable mood. Many children with DMDD also meet ODD criteria, making the distinction murky. However, ODD primarily involves oppositional behavior directed at authority figures, while DMDD includes explosive responses to frustration from any source—peers, siblings, or even the child's own performance. Additionally, the severity and frequency of outbursts tends to exceed typical ODD presentations. Some clinicians diagnose ODD when DMDD might be more accurate, particularly if they're unfamiliar with DMDD criteria.

ADHD with emotional dysregulation can look similar to DMDD. Children with ADHD often struggle with impulsivity and frustration tolerance, leading to emotional outbursts when things don't go their way. The key distinction lies in baseline irritability and outburst severity. Children with ADHD may have more emotional volatility than neurotypical children, but they don't typically maintain the pervasive, chronic irritability characteristic of DMDD. Many children have both conditions, further complicating diagnosis.

Anxiety disorders sometimes underlie irritability and behavioral outbursts. An anxious child might explode when facing a feared situation or when anxiety becomes overwhelming. However, anxiety-driven behavior typically links more directly to identifiable anxiety triggers, and the child shows clear signs of worry, fear, or avoidance. Children with DMDD may also have anxiety disorders, but the irritability and explosions occur across diverse situations not solely tied to anxiety.

Autism spectrum disorder can include emotional dysregulation, particularly around sensory sensitivities or changes in routine. Children with autism may have intense meltdowns that resemble DMDD outbursts. However, autism involves core features of social communication differences, restricted interests, and sensory processing differences that explain the behavioral responses. Careful evaluation distinguishes autism with co-occurring mood dysregulation from DMDD.

Intermittent explosive disorder (IED) involves sudden episodes of impulsive, aggressive outbursts. The distinction from DMDD centers on baseline mood. Children with IED return to normal mood between outbursts, while those with DMDD maintain chronic irritability. Additionally, DMDD cannot be diagnosed if IED better explains the symptoms— effectively, DMDD takes precedence in children showing chronic irritability plus outbursts.

Case Example: Sophie, Age 11

Sophie's diagnostic story illustrates how misdiagnosis delays appropriate treatment. At age seven, following her second suspension from school for throwing chairs during a rage episode, Sophie saw a child psychiatrist who diagnosed bipolar disorder. The psychiatrist noted Sophie's extreme mood swings and prescribed a mood stabilizer. Over six months, Sophie gained fifteen pounds and developed tremors but showed no behavioral improvement.

A second psychiatrist changed the diagnosis to ODD and recommended a behavioral intervention program focused on compliance training. Sophie completed the program but continued having frequent, severe outbursts. The third psychiatrist recognized ADHD and started stimulant medication, which helped Sophie's attention and impulsivity but didn't touch the irritability or rages.

Finally, at age eleven, Sophie saw a psychiatrist who specialized in complex mood disorders. She spent two sessions gathering history, reviewed records from previous providers, and interviewed Sophie's parents and teachers. This psychiatrist explained that Sophie had both ADHD and DMDD—the ADHD affected her attention and impulsivity, while DMDD explained the chronic irritability and explosive outbursts. With accurate diagnosis, Sophie's treatment plan changed to address both conditions appropriately. Sophie's mother expressed frustration at the four lost years but also relief that someone finally understood her daughter's struggles accurately.

What to Expect During Evaluation

Comprehensive DMDD evaluation typically involves multiple components across several appointments. Understanding the process reduces anxiety and helps families prepare effectively.

Initial intake usually starts with a detailed clinical interview. The clinician will ask about current symptoms, including specific examples of outbursts, baseline mood, triggers, duration and frequency of episodes, and impact on daily functioning. They'll explore developmental history from pregnancy through present, asking about early temperament, developmental milestones, trauma or stressful events, medical history, and previous mental health treatment. Family psychiatric history matters—mental health conditions run in families, and knowing about depression, anxiety, bipolar disorder, ADHD, or substance abuse in relatives helps inform diagnostic thinking.

Behavioral observations occur during appointments, though clinicians recognize that children often behave differently in clinical settings than at home or school. Some children show their irritability and oppositional behavior during appointments. Others save their worst behavior for safe environments, appearing compliant and regulated in the office. Clinicians account for this by relying heavily on parent and teacher reports rather than solely on their direct observations.

Rating scales and questionnaires provide standardized data. Common tools include the Child Behavior Checklist (completed by parents and teachers), which assesses a broad range of emotional and behavioral problems; the Screen for Child Anxiety Related Emotional Disorders (SCARED), which identifies anxiety symptoms; and various ADHD rating scales. No validated screening tool exists specifically for DMDD yet, so clinicians use general scales assessing irritability, anger, aggression, and mood regulation.

Diagnostic interviews may include structured or semi-structured formats. Some clinicians use the Kiddie Schedule for Affective Disorders and Schizophrenia (K-SADS), a detailed interview that systematically assesses psychiatric disorders in children. This tool helps clinicians determine if a child meets full diagnostic criteria for DMDD and identify comorbid conditions.

Teacher input provides crucial information about functioning in school. Clinicians may request that parents have teachers complete rating scales or provide written descriptions of the child's behavior, peer interactions, academic performance, and response to structure and demands.

Ruling out other conditions involves considering medical problems that might mimic psychiatric symptoms. Sleep disorders, for instance, severely impact mood regulation. Chronic pain conditions can make children irritable. Certain medications have behavioral side effects. Substance use (even in relatively young children) can affect mood and behavior. Trauma history requires careful assessment, as trauma responses can include emotional dysregulation and explosive behavior.

Diagnostic clarification often takes time. After initial evaluation, the clinician may provide a working diagnosis but schedule follow-up appointments to monitor symptoms, gather additional information, or observe treatment response. Sometimes diagnosis becomes clearer over time or needs revision as new information emerges.

The evaluation process can feel intrusive and exhausting. You'll answer personal questions, describe your child's worst moments repeatedly, admit to parenting strategies that didn't work, and expose family vulnerabilities. But thorough evaluation leads to accurate diagnosis, which makes all the difference in accessing appropriate treatment and support.

Preparing for a Productive Evaluation

Families can take specific steps to make the diagnostic process as efficient and accurate as possible.

Document systematically before the appointment. Track outbursts for at least two weeks, noting date, time, trigger (if identifiable), duration, intensity, and what helped (if anything). Record baseline mood daily. Note any patterns—times of day, specific situations, or circumstances that seem to make things better or worse. Bring this documentation to appointments.

Gather records from previous healthcare providers, schools, therapists, or other professionals who've worked with your child. Sign release forms allowing your current evaluator to obtain records directly. Don't assume providers will communicate automatically—make it happen.

Write a timeline of your child's development, starting from pregnancy and birth. Note when symptoms first appeared, how they've changed over time, and any significant life events (moves, family changes, trauma, medical issues) that coincided with behavioral changes.

List all medications your child has tried, including dosages, duration, effects (both beneficial and adverse), and reasons for discontinuation. Include supplements, over-the-counter medications, and any alternative treatments.

Compile family psychiatric history for both parents' sides of the family. Mental health conditions, substance abuse, learning disabilities, and developmental disorders in relatives all provide useful genetic information.

Prepare your child age-appropriately. Explain that you're going to talk to a doctor who helps kids with big feelings and tough behaviors. Emphasize that the child isn't in trouble and that the goal is to help them feel better and have an easier time managing their emotions. Older children and teens can participate more directly in the evaluation process.

Be honest during interviews. Don't minimize symptoms out of fear of judgment or exaggerate to ensure providers take you seriously. Present information accurately and completely. If you don't know an answer, say so. If you disagree with your co-parent about something, acknowledge the disagreement.

Ask questions throughout the process. If you don't understand something the clinician says, ask for clarification. If recommendations seem unclear, ask for more details. If you're worried about a particular treatment approach, voice your concerns. Good clinicians welcome questions and see them as indicators of engaged, thoughtful parents.

The evaluation process marks a critical step toward getting your child help. While the journey can feel overwhelming, each step moves you closer to understanding, treatment, and ultimately, hope for improvement. Accurate diagnosis doesn't solve everything—the real work of treatment lies ahead—but it provides an essential foundation for moving forward.

Looking Ahead

Diagnosis gives your child's struggles a name and provides a framework for understanding behavior that previously seemed inexplicable. But naming the problem is just the beginning. The next phase involves exploring treatment options, understanding what research and clinical experience suggest works, making decisions about therapy and medications, and learning strategies to manage daily life with a child who experiences the world through a lens of persistent irritability. The treatment landscape for DMDD draws from multiple sources—established therapies adapted from related conditions, emerging protocols developed specifically for severe irritability, and practical management techniques refined by families learning what helps their unique child. That landscape is our next destination.

Key Points Worth Noting

- DMDD requires twelve months of severe temper outbursts (three or more weekly) plus chronic irritability across multiple settings

- Distinguishing DMDD from similar conditions (bipolar, ODD, ADHD, anxiety, autism) requires careful evaluation by experienced clinicians

- Common misdiagnoses occur due to symptom overlap and clinicians' limited familiarity with DMDD

- Comprehensive evaluation includes clinical interviews, standardized rating scales, teacher input, developmental history, and ruling out other conditions

- Families can prepare effectively by documenting symptoms, gathering records, creating developmental timelines, and being thorough and honest during evaluation

- Accurate diagnosis provides the foundation for accessing appropriate treatment but represents the beginning rather than the end of the intervention journey

Chapter 3: The Treatment Landscape

Treatment decisions for DMDD require balancing scientific evidence, clinical experience, practical constraints, and your child's individual needs. No single treatment works for every child with DMDD, and no magic intervention makes symptoms disappear overnight. Instead, effective treatment typically involves combining multiple approaches—therapy, possible medication, parent training, school supports, and lifestyle modifications—while accepting that progress happens gradually and setbacks occur along the way. This chapter maps the treatment options currently available, helping you understand what each approach offers, what research supports, and how different interventions work together.

Evidence-Based Therapies

Cognitive Behavioral Therapy (CBT) represents one of the most studied psychological interventions for childhood emotional and behavioral disorders. CBT operates on the principle that thoughts, feelings, and behaviors interconnect—changing one affects the others. For children with DMDD, CBT helps identify distorted thinking patterns that fuel irritability and explosive behavior, then teaches skills to challenge those thoughts and respond differently.

A child with DMDD might think, "My teacher hates me" when given constructive feedback on homework. This thought generates anger and defensiveness, leading to an outburst. CBT teaches the child to recognize the thought, question its accuracy, and consider alternatives: "My teacher is trying to help me improve" or "This feedback is about my work, not about me personally." With the thought shift, the emotional intensity decreases, making regulated behavior more possible.

CBT sessions typically include:

Psychoeducation about emotions, how they work, and how DMDD affects emotional processing. Children learn that everyone experiences anger, frustration, and irritability, but their nervous system processes these emotions more intensely.

Cognitive restructuring teaches children to identify negative automatic thoughts, evaluate evidence for and against those thoughts, and generate more balanced alternative thoughts. The therapist might help a child track situations that trigger outbursts, identify the thoughts that arise in those moments, and practice more helpful ways of interpreting events.

Behavioral activation addresses the tendency of irritable children to withdraw from activities or interactions, which perpetuates negative mood. The therapist helps identify activities the child enjoys and schedules regular engagement in those activities regardless of mood state.

Problem-solving skills help children address challenges more effectively rather than becoming overwhelmed and explosive. The therapist teaches a structured approach: identify the problem, generate possible solutions, evaluate pros and cons of each option, select one solution to try, implement it, and evaluate the outcome.

Frustration tolerance training gradually exposes children to mildly frustrating situations while teaching coping skills. The therapist might start with puzzles or games that include some challenge, helping the child practice staying regulated when things don't go perfectly.

Research shows that CBT reduces symptoms of anxiety and depression in children, and preliminary studies suggest benefits for irritability as well. However, traditional CBT assumes certain cognitive capacities—the ability to identify and articulate thoughts, engage in logical evaluation of evidence, and implement strategies independently. Younger children or those with cognitive limitations may need adapted approaches.

Case Example: Aaron, Age 12

Aaron started CBT after his DMDD diagnosis at age eleven. His therapist, Dr. Martinez, spent the first several sessions building rapport and teaching Aaron about his nervous system's tendency to react strongly to frustration. Using diagrams and metaphors, Dr. Martinez explained how Aaron's brain worked like a smoke alarm set too sensitively—detecting threats everywhere even when situations were actually safe.

In session four, they began identifying Aaron's thinking patterns. Dr. Martinez asked Aaron to describe recent outbursts in detail. One incident involved Aaron destroying his science project after receiving a B rather than an A. Dr. Martinez helped Aaron identify his automatic thoughts: "I'm stupid. I can't do anything right. Nothing I do is good enough." These thoughts amplified Aaron's disappointment to unbearable levels.

Over subsequent sessions, Aaron practiced challenging these thoughts. Dr. Martinez asked questions like: "Is getting a B evidence that you're stupid, or evidence that this particular project didn't go perfectly?" "Does one B mean you can't do anything right, or does it mean you're a human being who sometimes does B-level work?" "Whose standard are you trying to meet—is a B really not good enough, or are you setting an impossibly high bar?"

Aaron learned to generate alternative thoughts: "I did good work on this project. A B is a respectable grade. I'm disappointed, but disappointment is different from failure." With less catastrophic thinking, Aaron's emotional reaction to setbacks became more manageable. The work took six months of weekly sessions plus homework assignments, but Aaron's outburst frequency decreased from five weekly to two weekly, and the intensity lessened.

Dialectical Behavior Therapy adapted for Children (DBT-C) builds on CBT principles but focuses more intensively on emotion regulation skills. Originally developed by Marsha Linehan for adults with severe emotion dysregulation, DBT was adapted for adolescents and, more recently, for younger children. DBT-C addresses DMDD particularly well because it directly targets the core problem: difficulty regulating intense emotions.

DBT-C teaches four skill modules:

Mindfulness trains children to stay present with their current experience rather than getting caught in rumination about the past or worry about the future. For children with DMDD, mindfulness practice helps them notice emotions arising without immediately reacting. A child learns to observe, "I'm feeling angry right now" rather than being completely consumed by the anger.

Distress tolerance provides skills for managing intense emotional distress without making the situation worse. Children learn radical acceptance (accepting reality as it is rather than fighting against it), self-soothing techniques (using senses to calm themselves), and distraction strategies (temporarily shifting attention from the trigger). When a child with DMDD faces an unchangeable frustration—a cancelled playdate due to weather, for instance—distress tolerance skills help them accept reality and cope rather than exploding.

Emotion regulation teaches strategies for understanding emotions, reducing vulnerability to emotional dysregulation, and changing unwanted emotions. Children learn to identify and label emotions accurately, understand what function emotions serve, and take steps to shift emotional states when helpful. They also learn to increase positive emotional experiences and build resilience.

Interpersonal effectiveness focuses on maintaining relationships while still getting needs met and maintaining self-respect. Children learn to ask for what they need assertively without aggression, say no effectively, and handle interpersonal conflict without exploding. For children with DMDD who often damage relationships through explosive behavior, these skills prove critical.

DBT-C typically involves weekly individual therapy, a weekly skills group, phone coaching between sessions (the therapist remains available for brief calls when the child needs help using skills in real situations), and consultation team meetings for therapists. The comprehensive approach requires significant commitment from families and therapists but shows strong evidence for reducing self-harm and suicidal behavior in adolescents with severe emotion dysregulation.

Case Example: Isabel, Age 10

Isabel's explosive outbursts included self-harm—hitting her head against walls, scratching her arms until they bled, and pulling out her hair. Her therapist recommended DBT-C after CBT proved insufficient. Isabel attended individual therapy weekly and a skills group with five other children struggling with emotional regulation.

The skills group taught one module every eight weeks, cycling through mindfulness, distress tolerance, emotion regulation, and interpersonal effectiveness. Isabel learned to use the "TIPP" skill for immediate crisis—Temperature (using cold water to calm her nervous system), Intense exercise (doing jumping jacks to burn off adrenaline), Paced breathing (slowing her breath to shift from fight-or-flight to calm), and Progressive muscle relaxation. When Isabel felt an explosion building, she practiced excusing herself to the bathroom to splash cold water on her face and breathe deeply for sixty seconds.

The emotion regulation module helped Isabel understand that she felt emotions more intensely than her peers—like her emotional volume knob stayed permanently turned to eight out of ten. She learned to reduce her vulnerability to emotional explosion by prioritizing sleep, eating regular meals, getting physical activity, and treating physical illness promptly. These basics sounded simple but made significant differences in Isabel's baseline irritability.

After eighteen months of DBT-C, Isabel's self-harm stopped completely, and her explosive outbursts decreased by approximately 60 percent. She still had DMDD—she remained more irritable than her peers—but she'd developed tools to manage the intensity and regulate herself more effectively.

Parent Training Programs recognize that parents need specialized skills to respond effectively to DMDD. These programs teach caregivers how to anticipate triggers, structure the environment to reduce explosions, respond during outbursts in ways that promote regulation rather than escalation, and reinforce positive behavior systematically.

Parent Management Training (PMT), developed by Alan Kazdin at Yale, provides one well-researched approach. PMT focuses on:

Positive attending teaches parents to notice and comment on appropriate behavior rather than only paying attention when behavior is problematic. Children with DMDD receive overwhelmingly negative feedback because their behavior creates constant problems. PMT helps parents deliberately catch their child being good, offering specific praise: "I noticed you took a deep breath instead of yelling when your sister touched your toy. That took real self-control."

Strategic use of consequences employs both rewards for positive behavior and nonphysical, logical consequences for problematic behavior. Parents learn to implement time-outs effectively (brief, immediate, and consistent), use privilege removal, and establish clear behavior-consequence connections.

Antecedent control involves identifying situations that commonly trigger outbursts and modifying those situations to prevent explosions. If homework battles occur daily, antecedent control might involve breaking work into smaller chunks, providing movement breaks, or changing the time or location of homework.

Problem-solving training helps families address ongoing behavioral challenges systematically rather than reacting emotionally and inconsistently. Parents learn to define problems specifically, generate multiple possible solutions, evaluate options, implement one solution, and adjust based on results.

Research demonstrates that PMT reduces oppositional behavior, aggression, and noncompliance in children with various disruptive behavior disorders. For DMDD specifically, parent training helps reduce environmental triggers and improve parent-child interactions, though it doesn't eliminate the underlying mood dysregulation.

Case Example: The Martinez Family

James and Elena Martinez enrolled in a ten-session PMT program at their therapist's recommendation. Their son Carlos, age eight, had multiple daily outbursts that left the family exhausted and disconnected. The first sessions focused on observation—James and Elena tracked situations preceding Carlos's outbursts and identified patterns. Homework time, transitions between activities, and situations involving perceived unfairness triggered most explosions.

The therapist taught James and Elena to prevent rather than react. They implemented a visual schedule so Carlos knew what came next, reducing transition-related outbursts. They broke homework into ten-minute segments with movement breaks between segments, addressing the homework trigger. They established a "complaint box" where Carlos could write down things that felt unfair, which Elena and James reviewed daily, acknowledging his feelings and problem-solving when possible.

The program also taught James and Elena to reward Carlos's use of coping skills rather than only focusing on outcomes. Previously, they'd respond angrily when Carlos exploded but ignore when he managed frustration successfully. After PMT, they actively noticed: "Carlos, you were really frustrated when you lost that game, but you didn't throw the pieces. I saw you take some deep breaths. That's using your skills." This positive attention increased Carlos's motivation to keep trying regulation strategies.

By program end, the Martinez family reported more positive interactions, fewer daily explosions, and greater confidence in their parenting. Carlos still had DMDD—his irritability hadn't disappeared—but the family functioned better together.

The Matthews Protocol Explained

The Matthews Protocol represents an emerging medication approach developed specifically for severe irritability and explosive outbursts characteristic of DMDD. Dr. Dan Matthews spent decades researching causes and treatments for severe explosive behavior in children, developing a medication combination that targets the neurobiological underpinnings of these symptoms.

The protocol uses two medications:

Amantadine, originally developed as an antiviral medication and later found helpful for Parkinson's disease, affects dopamine neurotransmission. In DMDD, amantadine appears to help reduce irritability and improve frustration tolerance. The medication carries relatively mild side effects compared to many psychiatric medications—dizziness, insomnia, and nausea occur in some children but typically resolve or improve with dosage adjustment.

Oxcarbazepine (Trileptal), an anti-seizure medication also used as a mood stabilizer, helps regulate neural excitability. In DMDD, it appears to reduce explosive outbursts and stabilize baseline mood. Side effects can include drowsiness, dizziness, and low sodium levels (which requires occasional blood test monitoring).

The Matthews Protocol implements these medications sequentially rather than simultaneously, allowing identification of each medication's effects and side effects separately. Treatment typically starts with amantadine at low doses, gradually increasing to therapeutic levels over several weeks. After amantadine reaches an effective dose, oxcarbazepine is introduced similarly.

Preliminary reports from psychiatrists using the Matthews Protocol suggest success rates exceeding 75 percent in reducing outbursts and improving irritability. Families describe dramatic improvements—children who previously exploded daily having several calm weeks, irritable children showing more positive baseline moods, families able to engage in normal activities that were impossible before. However, important caveats exist. Large-scale controlled research trials haven't yet been published. The protocol represents off-label use of both medications— they're FDA-approved for other conditions but not specifically for DMDD. Not every child responds, and some children experience problematic side effects requiring discontinuation.

Additionally, the protocol requires careful implementation and monitoring by psychiatrists experienced with this approach.

Case Example: Nathan, Age 9

Nathan's family had tried multiple medications before discovering the Matthews Protocol. Stimulants helped his ADHD but didn't touch his irritability. Antidepressants provided minimal benefit with significant side effects. Low-dose antipsychotics reduced explosive intensity somewhat but caused weight gain and sedation that Nathan's parents found unacceptable.

Nathan's psychiatrist, familiar with the Matthews Protocol, suggested trying this approach. They started amantadine at 25 mg each morning, increasing by 25 mg every five days until Nathan reached 100 mg daily. Within three weeks, Nathan's parents noticed improved frustration tolerance. Nathan still got angry when things didn't go his way, but the anger didn't escalate to explosive levels as quickly. His baseline mood improved slightly—still more irritable than typical children, but less perpetually grumpy.

After six weeks on amantadine alone, the psychiatrist added oxcarbazepine, starting at 150 mg twice daily and increasing gradually to 450 mg twice daily over four weeks. The addition of oxcarbazepine produced more dramatic changes. Nathan's explosive outbursts, which had occurred four to six times weekly before medication, dropped to once weekly or less. His mood improved further. Teachers reported Nathan seemed more engaged and less cranky. Siblings noted they could interact with Nathan without constant worry about triggering an explosion.

Nathan remained on the Matthews Protocol for two years, with periodic dosage adjustments as he grew. The medications didn't cure his DMDD—he still had more emotional intensity than typical children—but they reduced symptoms enough that therapy could work effectively and family life became manageable. Nathan's parents considered the treatment transformative.

Medication Options: Benefits, Risks, and Realities

Beyond the Matthews Protocol, psychiatrists prescribe various medications for DMDD, adapted from treatments used for related conditions. No medications carry FDA approval specifically for DMDD, making all use technically "off-label."

Stimulant medications (methylphenidate, amphetamine preparations) primarily treat ADHD but research suggests they also reduce irritability in some children with DMDD. Stimulants increase dopamine and norepinephrine activity, improving attention, impulse control, and frustration tolerance. Side effects include appetite suppression, sleep difficulties, possible mood changes, and in rare cases, increased anxiety or irritability. Many children with DMDD also have ADHD, making stimulants a logical first medication choice.

Antidepressants, particularly selective serotonin reuptake inhibitors (SSRIs), help some children with DMDD. Medications like sertraline, fluoxetine, and escitalopram increase serotonin availability, which can improve mood regulation and reduce irritability. One small study suggested combining an SSRI with a stimulant provided benefits for irritability. Side effects include gastrointestinal upset, behavioral activation or sedation, and rare but serious increased risk of suicidal thinking (requiring careful monitoring, especially when starting medication or changing doses).

Atypical antipsychotics (risperidone, aripiprazole) reduce severe aggression and explosive behavior effectively. These medications affect dopamine and serotonin systems, damping down emotional reactivity and impulsivity. They show the strongest evidence for reducing severe irritability and aggression but carry the most concerning side effects—significant weight gain, metabolic changes (increased blood sugar and cholesterol), movement abnormalities, and sedation. Psychiatrists typically reserve atypical antipsychotics for cases where other approaches have failed and severe behavior threatens the child's safety or family stability.

Alpha-2 agonists (guanfacine, clonidine), originally blood pressure medications, also help ADHD symptoms and can reduce irritability. These medications calm the sympathetic nervous system, reducing physiological arousal. Side effects include sedation, low blood pressure, and dizziness.

Mood stabilizers like lithium or valproate, commonly used for bipolar disorder, show mixed results for DMDD. Some children respond well, others show minimal benefit. Side effects vary by medication but can include weight gain, cognitive dulling, tremors, and need for regular blood monitoring.

The reality of medication treatment for DMDD involves trial and error. Psychiatrists make educated guesses about which medications might help based on symptom profile, co-occurring conditions, side effect concerns, and their clinical experience. A medication that works brilliantly for one child might provide zero benefit or cause intolerable side effects in another child. Finding the right medication or medication combination often requires trying multiple options over months or years.

Medications also don't work in isolation. They function best as part of comprehensive treatment including therapy, parent training, school supports, and lifestyle modifications. Even highly effective medications reduce rather than eliminate symptoms. A child might go from having five explosive outbursts weekly to one weekly—huge improvement, but still challenging.

Integrative Approaches

Some families explore treatments beyond conventional psychiatry and psychology, seeking integrative approaches that address nutrition, sleep, exercise, stress reduction, and alternative therapies.

Nutritional interventions focus on how diet affects mood and behavior. Some children show sensitivity to certain foods, with behavioral worsening after consuming particular ingredients. Common targets include food dyes, preservatives, sugar, gluten, and dairy. Limited research supports dietary interventions for DMDD specifically, but some families report improvements. Trying elimination diets requires careful implementation with professional guidance to ensure nutritional adequacy.

Sleep optimization proves critical. Insufficient or poor-quality sleep significantly worsens mood dysregulation. Establishing consistent bedtime routines, ensuring age-appropriate sleep duration (nine to twelve hours for school-age children), addressing sleep disorders (sleep apnea, restless legs syndrome), and creating conducive sleep environments all support better emotional regulation.

Regular physical activity helps regulate mood through multiple mechanisms—reducing stress hormones, increasing endorphins, improving sleep, providing structured outlets for energy. Children with DMDD benefit from daily physical activity, though team sports may prove challenging given their interpersonal difficulties. Individual activities like swimming, martial arts, or cycling might work better.

Omega-3 fatty acids (fish oil supplements) show evidence for improving mood in some psychiatric conditions. The mechanism likely involves reducing neural inflammation and supporting brain cell membrane function. While research specifically for

DMDD is limited, omega-3 supplementation is generally safe and might provide modest benefits.

Magnesium supplementation addresses potential deficiency that could worsen mood dysregulation. Magnesium plays roles in nervous system function and stress response. Some clinicians recommend supplementation, particularly for children with inadequate dietary intake.

Mindfulness and yoga practices teach self-regulation skills through body awareness and breath control. These practices help children notice emotional arousal early and implement calming strategies before reaching explosion. Programs designed specifically for children make these practices accessible and engaging.

Neurofeedback trains children to modify brain wave patterns associated with emotional dysregulation. While some practitioners and families report benefits, research evidence remains mixed and insurance typically doesn't cover this expensive treatment.

Parents considering integrative approaches should discuss plans with their child's healthcare team, ensure treatments don't interfere with conventional care, watch for concerning side effects, and maintain realistic expectations. Some integrative approaches provide genuine benefits, others prove ineffective, and a few might cause harm. Careful evaluation and monitoring protect children while allowing families to explore options that align with their values and goals.

Treatment for DMDD draws from many sources precisely because the condition is complex and newly recognized. The most effective approach typically combines multiple interventions tailored to your child's needs, your family's circumstances, and practical considerations like insurance coverage and local treatment availability. Finding what works requires patience, persistence, and willingness to adjust course when particular approaches prove ineffective. But effective treatment exists, and most children with DMDD improve significantly with appropriate, comprehensive intervention.

Building the Foundation

Treatment doesn't happen in isolation from daily life. The therapies, medications, and interventions described here provide tools and support, but families still face the day-to-day reality of living with a child who struggles with emotional regulation. The next chapter shifts focus to practical strategies for managing daily life—identifying what triggers your child's explosions, learning techniques to prevent or de-escalate outbursts, creating systems and tools that promote regulation, and knowing when situations require emergency intervention. These practical skills transform treatment concepts into lived experience, making theoretical knowledge operational in your actual family life.

Essential Points to Carry Forward

- No single treatment cures DMDD; effective intervention typically combines therapy, possible medication, parent training, and supports

- CBT helps children identify and modify distorted thinking patterns that fuel emotional explosions

- DBT-C directly teaches emotion regulation skills including mindfulness, distress tolerance, and interpersonal effectiveness

- Parent training programs equip caregivers with specialized strategies for preventing triggers and responding effectively to dysregulated behavior

- The Matthews Protocol (amantadine plus oxcarbazepine) shows promising preliminary results with over 75% success rates in reducing severe irritability and outbursts

- Various medications provide options when first choices prove ineffective, though all use for DMDD is off-label and involves trial-and-error

- Integrative approaches including nutrition, sleep optimization, exercise, and supplements may complement conventional treatment for some children

- Treatment requires patience—finding effective interventions often takes months of trying different approaches and combinations

Chapter 4: Daily Life Management

The crisis happens on a Wednesday morning before school. Your child announces their blue shirt "feels wrong"—something about the tag, the fabric, the way it sits on their shoulders. Within thirty seconds of your suggestion to try a different shirt, your child is screaming, throwing clothes, and sobbing that you never listen, you don't care, and their entire day is ruined. You're already running late, you have a meeting in an hour, and your child's breakdown shows no signs of stopping. This is real life with DMDD—not the clean treatment plans discussed in therapy sessions, but the moment-by-moment, exhausting work of helping your child get through a day without melting down or maintaining your own composure when they do.

Identifying Triggers and Patterns

Children with DMDD explode frequently enough that parents might assume triggers are random or that the child is simply "bad" or willfully defiant. In reality, most explosions follow identifiable patterns, though recognizing those patterns requires systematic observation because stress and exhaustion cloud memory and perception.

Start tracking triggers immediately. Use a simple format—date, time, what happened right before the explosion, what the child was doing, who was present, what the explosion looked like (verbal, physical, duration), and what helped (if anything). Track every outburst for at least two weeks, preferably four. Patterns emerge that single incidents hide.

Common trigger categories include:

Transitions between activities, locations, or expectations disrupt children with DMDD particularly powerfully. Moving from preferred activities to non-preferred activities (stopping video games for homework) causes obvious difficulties, but even neutral transitions (finishing breakfast to get dressed, moving from math to reading at school) can trigger explosions. The cognitive shifting required for transitions taxes executive function, and children with DMDD have less capacity for managing that additional demand.

Frustration related to tasks that feel difficult, confusing, or failure-prone provokes explosions. Homework in subjects the child finds challenging becomes a nightly battlefield. Losing games triggers rage. Making errors on assignments leads to destroyed papers and refusal to continue. The child's low frustration tolerance means that typical learning challenges escalate immediately rather than prompting problem-solving.

Sensory experiences affect some children with DMDD significantly. Clothing tags, certain fabric textures, bright lights, loud noises, strong smells, food textures, or being touched unexpectedly can shift a child from baseline irritability to explosion. These sensory triggers operate differently from autism-related sensory processing differences—the child isn't necessarily sensory-seeking or sensory-avoiding across the board, but specific sensory experiences in certain states (when already stressed or tired) become unbearable.

Perceived unfairness or rejection triggers intense reactions. A sibling getting slightly more juice, a friend choosing someone else to partner with, a parent appearing to favor another child— all generate explosive responses. The child interprets ambiguous situations negatively, assuming hostility or rejection even when none exists.

Hunger, fatigue, illness, and pain amplify baseline irritability and reduce the child's capacity to manage frustration. A child who might tolerate a minor frustration when rested and fed explodes over the same frustration when hungry or tired. Physical states matter enormously.

Overstimulation from too much activity, too many people, too much noise, or too many demands depletes the child's regulatory capacity. Birthday parties, family gatherings, field trips, or even unusually busy school days often end in explosions—not because the activities themselves were terrible, but because the cumulative stimulation exceeded the child's ability to cope.

Unpredictability and lack of control leave children with DMDD feeling unsafe and anxious. Surprises—even positive ones—can trigger explosions because they disrupt the child's sense of knowing what to expect. Schedule changes, unexpected visitors, or spontaneous plans cause dysregulation.

Case Example: The Thompson Family's Discovery

Rebecca Thompson tracked her daughter Lily's outbursts for three weeks before patterns emerged. Initially, Rebecca thought triggers were random—Lily seemed to explode over nothing. But the tracking revealed clear patterns:

1. **After-school explosions**: Lily exploded within thirty minutes of arriving home from school on fourteen of fifteen school days. The specific trigger varied (homework, snack not being ready, sibling interaction), but the timing was consistent.

2. **Weekend afternoon meltdowns**: Saturday and Sunday afternoons around 2 PM saw explosions seven of six weekend days. Rebecca realized this coincided with low blood sugar—Lily often skipped or ate minimal lunch on weekends while playing.

3. **Morning clothing battles**: Monday, Wednesday, and Friday mornings involved clothing-related explosions. Rebecca noticed these were gym days when Lily had to bring extra clothing to school, adding complexity to the morning routine.

4. **Transition-related rages**: Any transition generated potential for explosion, but certain transitions—finishing screen time, ending preferred activities, moving to homework—caused explosions ninety percent of the time.

Recognizing these patterns allowed Rebecca to implement preventive strategies. She built in thirty minutes of decompression time after school before making any demands on Lily. She ensured Lily ate lunch on weekends by setting alarms and providing preferred foods. She prepared gym clothes the night before on those mornings. She gave five-minute, three-minute, and one-minute warnings before transitions. These changes didn't eliminate Lily's explosions, but they reduced frequency from fourteen weekly to six weekly—still challenging, but significantly more manageable.

De-Escalation Techniques That Actually Work

Once a child with DMDD begins escalating toward explosion, parents have a narrow window to intervene effectively. The techniques that work depend on how far into the escalation cycle the child has progressed.

Early escalation shows in subtle signs—increased body tension, facial expression changes, voice tone shifts, reduced frustration tolerance, and minor irritability. At this stage, prevention strategies can still work:

Environmental modification reduces demands and stimulation immediately. If you notice your child starting to escalate during homework, implementing a break prevents full explosion. If irritability increases during sibling interaction, separating the children heads off the crisis.

Co-regulation through calm presence helps some children. Moving physically closer (if the child tolerates proximity when upset), using a calm voice, and providing simple choices ("Do you want to take a break in your room or on the couch?") sometimes stops escalation. Your own regulation matters here— if you're anxious or frustrated, your child picks up those emotions and escalates further.

Redirection to a calming activity works if the child isn't too far into escalation. Suggesting they get a drink of water, step outside for fresh air, listen to music, or engage in a favored calming activity can shift their trajectory.

Validation acknowledges the child's feeling without agreeing that their reaction is proportionate. "You're really frustrated that you have to do homework right now. I get that homework is hard sometimes." This validation helps the child feel understood rather than dismissed.

Mid-escalation involves louder voice, more intense body language, verbal aggression (yelling, threatening), and possibly minor physical aggression (throwing soft objects, slamming doors). At this stage, prevention has failed and de-escalation requires different approaches:

Stop making demands immediately. Whatever you were asking the child to do no longer matters. Continuing to insist that they do homework, clean their room, or apologize will only escalate the situation further. You can return to the original issue later, but right now, the priority is preventing explosion.

Increase space between you and the child unless they specifically seek closeness. Many children need physical distance when escalating. Back away slowly, remain visible but not hovering, and give them room.

45

Reduce stimulation by lowering lights, reducing noise, removing siblings or other people from the immediate area, and minimizing sensory input. The child's nervous system is overwhelmed, and additional stimulation worsens their state.

Use minimal language. Long explanations, reasoning, or attempts to talk the child through their feelings typically backfire during escalation. Short, simple statements work better: "You're safe." "I'm going to stay nearby." "You can have space."

Full explosion involves intense verbal and/or physical aggression—screaming, throwing objects, hitting, kicking, destroying property, or self-harm. At this point, de-escalation isn't possible. The child's nervous system has fully activated fight-or-flight response, and they can't access rational thinking or regulatory strategies. Your goals shift to safety and allowing the storm to pass:

Ensure safety first. Remove dangerous objects if possible. Intervene physically only if the child is in immediate danger of serious injury (about to run into traffic, hurting themselves badly). If siblings are present, remove them from the situation—having them witness or be targeted by the explosion adds trauma for everyone.

Stay calm yourself. This is extraordinarily difficult when your child is raging, but your own escalation makes everything worse. Practice deep breathing, mentally recite a calming phrase, or focus on the knowledge that the explosion will end eventually.

Don't engage the content of what the child is yelling. If they're screaming that you're the worst parent ever and they hate you, don't defend yourself, don't argue, don't try to reason. The words come from a dysregulated nervous system, not from their true feelings.

Wait it out. Most explosions last fifteen to forty-five minutes before the intensity begins decreasing. You can't accelerate this process. You can only maintain safety and wait for the child's nervous system to exhaust itself.

Post-explosion requires careful handling. The child often feels exhausted, ashamed, or confused. Some children seek connection and comfort; others need continued space. Follow the child's lead:

Avoid immediate post-mortems. Trying to process what happened immediately after explosion usually triggers re-escalation. The child needs time to fully regulate before discussing the incident.

Provide physical comfort if the child seeks it—a hug, sitting together quietly, gentle touch. If they resist contact, offer proximity without touching.

Return to normal gradually. Once the child has calmed, slowly reintroduce typical expectations and routines. This might happen immediately or might require hours, depending on the severity of the explosion and the child's recovery pattern.

Process later. Several hours or even a day after explosion, you might help the child reflect on what happened, identify triggers, and practice alternative responses for the future. Some children benefit from this processing; others find it shaming and resist. Gauge your individual child's receptiveness.

Case Example: Learning What Works—The Garcia Family

Maria Garcia spent months trying to de-escalate her son Paulo's explosions using reasoning and explanation. When Paulo began escalating about homework, Maria would explain why homework mattered, offer to help, promise rewards for completion, and try to talk him into compliance. These attempts failed universally, usually worsening the explosion.

After working with a therapist who specialized in DMDD, Maria tried different approaches. When she noticed Paulo's early escalation signs—heavy sighs, pencil tapping, increasingly terse responses—she immediately suggested a movement break rather than explaining homework's importance. "Let's take five minutes. Go bounce on the trampoline or walk around the block." This early intervention prevented full explosion about sixty percent of the time.

When Paulo hit mid-escalation, Maria stopped all demands. "Never mind about homework right now. We'll figure that out later." This counterintuitive response felt like "giving in," but it consistently prevented escalation to full explosion.

When full explosion did occur, Maria learned to remove Paulo's siblings, secure any dangerous objects quickly, then position herself across the room where Paulo could see her but felt he had space. She stopped trying to reason with him during explosions. She breathed deeply, sometimes counting her breaths to stay calm, and waited. The explosions still happened and still felt terrible, but they became more predictable and slightly less intense as Maria stopped inadvertently fueling them with her own distress and engagement.

Creating a Regulation Toolbox

Children with DMDD need easily accessible strategies for managing emotional intensity before it reaches explosive levels. Creating a personalized toolbox of regulatory techniques gives children options when they feel themselves escalating.

Sensory strategies provide immediate input that can shift nervous system states:

Cold water on the face or hands activates the dive reflex, slowing heart rate and calming the nervous system. Some children benefit from splashing cold water on their face or holding ice cubes when escalating.

Intense physical activity burns adrenaline and provides proprioceptive input that regulates. Options include jumping jacks, running in place, push-ups against a wall, squeezing a stress ball, or jumping on a trampoline.

Deep pressure through weighted blankets, tight hugs, or being under heavy cushions provides calming input for some children.

Rhythmic activities like rocking, swinging, or bouncing on an exercise ball help regulate through predictable, repetitive movement.

Breathing techniques shift the nervous system from sympathetic (fight-or-flight) to parasympathetic (calm) activation:

Square breathing: Breathe in for four counts, hold for four counts, breathe out for four counts, hold for four counts. Repeat several times.

Belly breathing: Place a hand on the belly and breathe deeply enough that the hand rises and falls. This ensures diaphragmatic breathing rather than shallow chest breathing.

Counting breaths: Simply count each breath, focusing attention on the counting to break the cycle of rumination fueling emotional escalation.

Cognitive strategies learned through therapy can be distilled into quick techniques:

Thought-stopping: When catastrophic or angry thoughts spiral, the child practices saying "Stop!" internally or aloud, then deliberately shifts attention to something neutral or positive.

Positive self-talk: The child develops phrases that counter negative automatic thoughts. "I can handle this." "This feeling will pass." "I'm learning to manage my anger."

Perspective-taking: For older children, asking themselves "Will this matter in a day? A week? A year?" helps contextualize frustrations.

Distraction and redirection shift attention away from triggers:

Favorite activities: Having a go-to activity that's genuinely engaging and enjoyable provides escape when emotions become overwhelming. This might be drawing, building with LEGO, listening to specific music, watching particular videos, or playing with a pet.

Grounding exercises: Naming five things you can see, four things you can hear, three things you can touch, two things you can smell, and one thing you can taste brings attention into the present moment and out of emotional overwhelm.

Humor: For some families, appropriate humor can break tension. This requires careful calibration—making fun of the child's distress worsens things, but shared laughter about neutral topics can shift mood.

Environmental modifications create conditions that reduce regulatory demands:

Quiet space: Designating a room or corner where the child can go when overwhelmed provides a refuge. This isn't punishment—it's a tool. Making the space comfortable and equipped with calming items (soft lighting, comfortable seating, calming visuals, fidget toys) makes it more appealing.

Routine and predictability: Consistent daily schedules reduce anxiety and help the child know what to expect. Visual schedules showing the day's activities help children with DMDD feel more secure.

Reduced demands during vulnerable times: If tracking shows that after-school time is particularly volatile, that's not the time to make demands about homework, chores, or practicing instruments. Structure the day to minimize demands during high-risk times.

The toolbox requires teaching, practice, and patience. Children don't automatically use regulatory strategies when dysregulated. The strategies need to be taught during calm times, practiced repeatedly, and reinforced when used successfully. Many children initially resist using tools, insisting they don't work. With consistency and parental modeling (you using the same tools when you're stressed), most children eventually incorporate some strategies into their repertoire.

Case Example: Building Mia's Toolbox

Mia's parents worked with her therapist to identify regulation strategies that might help eight-year-old Mia. They tried multiple options, discovering that Mia responded well to cold water, intense exercise, and distraction but found breathing exercises frustrating and grounding techniques annoying.

They created a physical "toolbox"—actually a decorated container Mia kept in her room containing:

- A stress ball

- Ice packs (kept in the freezer for when needed)

- Cards listing activity choices (jump on trampoline, run around the house three times, do wall push-ups)

- Headphones and access to a calming music playlist

- A favorite fidget spinner

- Pictures of Mia's dog (who reliably made her smile)

During calm times, Mia's parents practiced using the toolbox with her. They role-played situations that might trigger escalation and practiced choosing and using tools. When Mia started showing early escalation signs, her parents prompted: "Time to use your toolbox. What might help right now?"

Initially, Mia refused or insisted nothing would help. Her parents stayed consistent, sometimes making specific suggestions: "Let's try the trampoline for two minutes." Over several months, Mia started using tools occasionally without prompting. When she did, her parents praised the effort regardless of outcome: "I noticed you used your stress ball when you felt yourself getting frustrated. That's using your skills."

A year into toolbox practice, Mia used regulatory strategies independently about thirty percent of the time when escalating. That thirty percent prevented many explosions and helped Mia feel more competent. The other seventy percent still required parental intervention, but the family felt encouraged by progress.

When to Seek Emergency Help

Most DMDD explosions, though exhausting and distressing, don't constitute emergencies. But certain situations require immediate professional intervention beyond your family's capacity to manage safely.

Seek emergency help when:

The child poses immediate danger to themselves. This includes serious self-harm (cutting with intent to cause significant injury, attempting to ingest harmful substances, trying to hurt themselves in ways that could cause lasting damage), suicidal statements that seem genuine rather than manipulative, or behaviors that could result in serious injury (running toward traffic, attempting to jump from dangerous heights).

The child poses immediate danger to others. While DMDD involves aggression, most aggressive behavior consists of hitting, kicking, or throwing objects that cause bruises but not serious injury. Emergency help becomes necessary when violence escalates to use of weapons, strangulation attempts, or assault causing or likely to cause significant harm.

You're losing control of your own responses. If you feel yourself approaching the point of harming your child physically in response to their behavior, you need immediate help. Call a crisis line, have another adult come to the house, or call emergency services. Your child's safety requires that you maintain control, and if that control is slipping, intervention is necessary.

The child experiences a psychiatric emergency. This includes first onset of psychotic symptoms (hallucinations, delusions, grossly disorganized thinking), extreme agitation lasting hours without any ability to calm, or complete inability to function requiring immediate psychiatric assessment.

You've exhausted all strategies and cannot maintain safety. Sometimes explosions persist so long or recur so frequently that parents reach the end of their capacity to manage. If you've tried all de-escalation techniques, implemented safety measures, and the situation continues escalating or hasn't resolved after several hours, professional help may be needed.

Options for emergency help include:

Mobile crisis teams dispatch to homes when families call, providing in-home assessment and intervention. These teams can sometimes prevent hospitalization by stabilizing situations and connecting families to services.

Emergency departments see children in psychiatric crisis. Be prepared for long waits, potentially traumatic experiences (emergency departments aren't designed for children), and possible recommendation for psychiatric hospitalization. Bring documentation of your child's diagnoses, medications, and recent behavioral history.

Crisis hotlines provide telephone support and can help you determine if your situation requires emergency services or can be managed with other interventions. The 988 Suicide and Crisis Lifeline operates nationwide.

Police involvement should be last resort when other options aren't available or safety is immediately threatened. Police officers typically lack training in mental health crisis intervention, and their presence can escalate situations. However, when a child is actively harming themselves seriously or others, and you cannot maintain safety, calling police may be necessary. Clearly state that this is a mental health crisis involving a child.

Psychiatric hospitalization provides intensive intervention when outpatient treatment proves insufficient and safety cannot be maintained at home. Hospitalizations typically last several days to two weeks, during which the team adjusts medications, teaches coping skills, ensures safety, and develops discharge plans. While hospitalization can be traumatic for children and families, it sometimes provides the reset needed to prevent tragedy and access more intensive treatment.

Case Example: When Things Became Too Dangerous

The Rodriguez family reached crisis point when eleven-year-old Antonio's explosions escalated to include choking his younger brother. In previous explosions, Antonio had hit, kicked, and thrown objects, causing bruises but nothing requiring medical attention. The choking incident lasted long enough that Antonio's brother lost consciousness briefly before Antonio's father pulled him off.

The family called 911. Police and ambulance responded. Antonio's brother was evaluated (he recovered fully) while police questioned the family. The crisis worker who accompanied police helped the family understand their options.

They could take Antonio to the emergency department for psychiatric evaluation. The hospital would likely admit him for stabilization and safety assessment.

The family made the difficult decision to take Antonio to the emergency department. After six hours in the ED, Antonio was admitted to the child psychiatric unit. He stayed nine days. During hospitalization, the psychiatrist adjusted Antonio's medications significantly, the social worker taught the family safety planning strategies, and Antonio participated in group therapy focusing on anger management.

Discharge planning included referrals to more intensive outpatient treatment, a crisis plan detailing steps to take if Antonio became dangerous again, and safety modifications at home (removing or locking up potential weapons, installing locks on sibling bedroom doors, identifying safe spaces for siblings during Antonio's explosions).

The hospitalization was traumatic for everyone but necessary. Antonio's behavior had exceeded what the family could manage safely at home. The intensive intervention prevented serious injury and connected the family to services they hadn't been able to access through outpatient channels.

Living with DMDD means developing skills you never imagined needing—tracking behavior patterns like a detective, de-escalating crises like a hostage negotiator, creating individualized intervention toolkits, and knowing when situations exceed your capacity to manage alone. These skills develop gradually through practice, mistakes, and small successes. No parent masters all these techniques immediately, and every family adapts approaches to fit their unique child and circumstances. But with persistence and support, daily life management becomes more predictable, explosions become less frequent or intense, and families find ways to function despite the ongoing challenges DMDD presents. The work continues beyond home, extending into the other major setting where children spend their days—school. That educational context presents its own challenges and requires specific strategies, which we'll address next.

Core Concepts for Daily Management

- Systematic tracking reveals trigger patterns invisible to stressed memory, enabling preventive intervention

- Common triggers include transitions, frustration, sensory experiences, perceived unfairness, physical states (hunger/fatigue), overstimulation, and unpredictability

- De-escalation techniques vary by escalation stage—early stage allows prevention, mid-stage requires stopping demands and increasing space, full explosion requires focusing solely on safety

- Regulation toolboxes provide children with accessible strategies including sensory input, breathing techniques, cognitive tools, distraction, and environmental modifications

- Tools require teaching during calm times, repeated practice, and consistent reinforcement when used

- Emergency help becomes necessary when children pose serious danger to self or others, parents lose control of responses, psychiatric emergencies occur, or families exhaust their capacity to maintain safety

- Options for crisis include mobile crisis teams, emergency departments, crisis hotlines, and (as last resort) police intervention

- Most DMDD challenges remain manageable at home with appropriate strategies, support, and gradually developing skills

Chapter 5: School Success Strategies

The call from school interrupts your work meeting. Your child destroyed another student's project during art class. The teacher used words like "unacceptable," "cannot tolerate," and "consequences." You'll need to pick up your child immediately—another suspension, the fourth this semester. You know your child didn't destroy the project maliciously. They became frustrated with their own project, spiraled into escalation, and lashed out at the nearest target. But the school sees only the behavior and its impact, not the neurological storm that drove it. Bridging this gap between understanding DMDD and maintaining educational access requires navigation skills, documentation prowess, and strategic advocacy.

Working with Teachers and Administrators

Teachers and administrators want to help students succeed but often lack specific training in managing DMDD. The disorder's recent introduction means most educators haven't encountered the diagnosis, don't understand how it differs from other disruptive behavior disorders, and feel uncertain about effective interventions. Your role involves educating, collaborating, and building partnerships that support your child's educational access.

Start with information sharing. Schedule a meeting specifically to discuss your child's diagnosis before major behavioral incidents force reactive rather than proactive planning. Bring documentation including a letter from your child's psychiatrist or psychologist explaining DMDD, how it manifests, what triggers to watch for, and recommended accommodations. Share articles or fact sheets about DMDD (organizations like CHADD and the Child Mind Institute offer free resources). Present this information as partnership: "I want to help you understand what's happening with my child so we can work together to support their success."

Explain the neuroscience in accessible terms. Help educators understand that children with DMDD aren't choosing defiant behavior—their nervous systems process frustration and disappointment differently. Use analogies: "Imagine your smoke alarm going off every time you make toast. That's how my child's brain works with frustration—minor irritations trigger major alarm responses, and they struggle to turn off the alarm." This reframing shifts understanding from willful misbehavior to neurological challenge requiring support rather than punishment.

Identify specific manifestations of DMDD in the classroom. General information about the disorder helps, but teachers need to know how DMDD looks in your particular child. Does your child shut down and refuse to work when frustrated, or explode verbally and disrupt the class? Do they struggle more during transitions, independent work time, or group activities? Does irritability show up as complaints, negative comments, or withdrawal? Specific descriptions help teachers recognize early escalation and intervene preventively.

Collaborate on strategies rather than dictating what teachers must do. Teachers possess expertise about classroom management and have to balance your child's needs against twenty to thirty other students. Ask what they've noticed works well. Share what helps at home. Problem-solve together: "Math homework causes major explosions at home. What happens during math class? Could we try breaking assignments into smaller chunks to reduce overwhelm?"

Acknowledge teacher challenges explicitly. Teaching a child with DMDD is genuinely difficult. Explosive behavior disrupts class, frightens other students, and exhausts teachers. Acknowledging these realities builds goodwill: "I know my child's behavior makes your job harder. I appreciate your willingness to keep working with us to find solutions."

Maintain regular communication through whatever method works for the teacher—email, weekly phone calls, communication notebook. Regular contact allows you to celebrate successes ("I heard my child participated well in group work today—thank you for that accommodation!"), address small problems before they become big ones, and maintain a relationship beyond crisis management.

Case Example: The Parker Family's Collaborative Approach

When seven-year-old Sam Parker started second grade with a new teacher, his parents Karen and Tom requested a meeting two weeks into the school year. Sam had been diagnosed with DMDD the previous spring but hadn't disclosed this to the new teacher yet. Karen and Tom brought a one-page handout about DMDD, a letter from Sam's psychiatrist, and a folder of work samples from the previous year showing what Sam could accomplish when regulated versus when dysregulated.

During the meeting, Karen explained: "Sam has a condition called Disruptive Mood Dysregulation Disorder. His brain processes frustration and disappointment differently than other kids. What might seem like a minor irritation to other children can feel overwhelming to Sam, and he hasn't yet developed good skills to manage those feelings." She described Sam's specific patterns—shutting down during challenging math work, becoming verbally aggressive when corrected, and needing movement breaks to maintain regulation.

The teacher, Ms. Johnson, shared that she'd noticed Sam seemed more irritable than other students and had already been giving him some extra processing time. Together, they developed a plan: Sam would have a "break card" he could use to take three-minute walks in the hallway when feeling overwhelmed. Ms. Johnson would check in with Sam privately when she noticed him getting frustrated, offering a choice of working with her support or taking a break. She'd break longer assignments into sections with check-ins between each section. She'd avoid calling attention to Sam's irritability in front of classmates.

Karen established weekly Friday afternoon email check-ins. Ms. Johnson sent brief summaries of the week's successes and challenges. Karen responded with thanks and suggestions for addressing challenges. This communication allowed them to adjust strategies based on what was working. By mid-year, Sam's explosive incidents decreased from weekly to monthly, and his academic performance improved as he spent more time engaged and less time dysregulated.

IEP vs. 504 Plans: What You Need to Know

Children with DMDD often qualify for educational supports under federal law. Two mechanisms provide these protections—Individualized Education Programs (IEPs) under the Individuals with Disabilities Education Act (IDEA) and 504 Plans under Section 504 of the Rehabilitation Act. Understanding differences helps you pursue appropriate protections for your child.

504 Plans provide accommodations for students with disabilities that affect major life activities, including learning. To qualify, a child must have a documented disability but doesn't need to require specialized instruction. The 504 Plan lists accommodations (modifications to how curriculum is delivered or how the student demonstrates learning) that allow the student to access education equally with peers. Examples include extended time on tests, preferential seating, frequent breaks, reduced homework load, or alternative spaces for testing.

504 Plans offer advantages of relatively simple implementation, fewer meetings, and flexibility to make quick accommodation adjustments. Limitations include no funding attached (schools aren't reimbursed for providing 504 accommodations), no specialized instruction provided, and fewer procedural protections if disputes arise.

IEPs serve students with disabilities who require specialized instruction—not just accommodations but actual modified teaching approaches to access curriculum. IEP qualification requires that the child has one of thirteen disability categories specified in IDEA (emotional disturbance, other health impairment, or specific learning disability most commonly apply to DMDD students) and that the disability adversely affects educational performance such that the child needs specialized instruction.

IEPs are comprehensive documents including present levels of academic achievement and functional performance, measurable annual goals, specialized instruction and related services, accommodations and modifications, participation with non-disabled peers, and transition planning for older students. Schools receive federal funding for students with IEPs, creating financial incentive to provide services. Parents have extensive procedural rights including participation in all meetings, consent requirements for changes, access to mediation and due process if disputes arise, and independent educational evaluation rights.

IEPs offer more comprehensive support and stronger protections but require more complex implementation, formal annual review meetings, and frequent documentation. Schools sometimes resist IEP qualification due to cost and procedural requirements.

Determining which to pursue depends on your child's needs. If your child can access curriculum with accommodations (extra time, breaks, modified presentation) but doesn't need different teaching methods, 504 might suffice. If your child requires specialized instruction (social skills training, behavior intervention plans, counseling services, modified curriculum), pursue an IEP. Some families start with 504, then advocate for IEP if needs exceed accommodations.

Both plans protect students from discipline for behavior related to their disability. Under IDEA, students with IEPs can't be suspended for more than ten cumulative days per year for disability-related behavior without triggering manifestation determination (formal evaluation of if behavior was caused by disability). 504 Plans provide similar protections though with less explicit procedures. This matters significantly for DMDD students who often face discipline for explosive behavior directly related to their disability.

Case Example: From 504 to IEP—Jasmine's Story

Jasmine qualified for a 504 Plan in third grade after her DMDD diagnosis. The plan included preferential seating near the teacher, five-minute movement breaks every thirty minutes, extended time on tests, and ability to complete tests in a quiet location. These accommodations helped moderately—Jasmine's behavior improved slightly but she still had weekly explosions and falling academic performance.

By fourth grade, Jasmine's parents requested IEP evaluation. The school initially resisted, arguing that Jasmine had passing grades and 504 accommodations were working. Jasmine's parents pushed back, providing documentation from Jasmine's psychiatrist that she required more intensive intervention than accommodations alone could provide. They highlighted that Jasmine had been suspended three times first semester for explosive behavior and was achieving Cs and Ds rather than the

As and Bs she'd earned in earlier grades before DMDD symptoms intensified.

The school conducted evaluations showing that Jasmine qualified under "emotional disturbance" category—her emotional and behavioral functioning significantly impaired her educational performance despite average cognitive abilities. The IEP team developed a comprehensive plan including:

Specialized instruction: Weekly sessions with the school counselor teaching emotion regulation skills, daily check-ins with a behavior intervention specialist who helped Jasmine implement strategies before escalation, and modified social studies and English assignments to reduce frustration while maintaining academic rigor.

Related services: Thirty minutes weekly of individual counseling with the school psychologist, monthly consultation between Jasmine's teacher and the school behavioral specialist, and crisis intervention support from the behavioral specialist when Jasmine began escalating.

Behavior intervention plan: Detailed plan identifying triggers, early warning signs, preventive strategies, de-escalation techniques, and teaching replacement behaviors (asking for breaks instead of exploding, using calming strategies independently).

Accommodations: Continued 504 accommodations plus additional ones including reduced homework load to prevent after-school explosions and permission to step out of class with a trusted adult when needed.

Goals: Measurable goals around Jasmine reducing explosive outbursts from weekly to twice monthly, independently using three calming strategies without prompting, and completing work at grade level in core subjects.

The IEP implementation took several months to show results but eventually made significant differences. The specialized instruction taught Jasmine skills beyond what accommodations alone could provide. The related services gave her consistent support. By year's end, Jasmine's explosive incidents decreased to monthly, her grades improved to mostly Bs, and she reported feeling more successful at school.

Specific Classroom Accommodations

Effective accommodations reduce environmental barriers to learning without lowering educational standards. For DMDD students, accommodations address emotion regulation challenges, frustration intolerance, difficulty with transitions, and interpersonal struggles.

Environmental accommodations modify the physical or social environment:

- Preferential seating near teacher for easy check-ins and monitoring

- Seating away from distractions (windows, doors, high-traffic areas)

- Access to alternative seating (standing desk, wobble stool, beanbag chair) for movement needs

- Designated quiet space in classroom or elsewhere for de-escalation

- Reduced visual clutter in work area to minimize overstimulation

Schedule and routine accommodations provide predictability and reduce transition stress:

- Visual schedule showing daily activities and any changes

- Advance notice of schedule changes when possible

- Five-minute, two-minute, and one-minute warnings before transitions
- Extra time for transitions between activities or locations
- Modified schedule if full school day proves overwhelming (shortened day, built-in breaks)

Assignment accommodations reduce frustration related to academic work:

- Breaking long assignments into shorter segments with breaks between
- Extended time to complete work without time pressure escalating stress
- Reduced homework load (fewer problems demonstrating same concept)
- Alternative demonstration of knowledge (verbal explanation instead of written report, drawing instead of essay)
- Use of assistive technology (computer for writing if handwriting causes frustration, calculator if arithmetic triggers explosions)

Testing accommodations address test anxiety and frustration:

- Extended time on tests and exams
- Testing in separate, quiet location
- Ability to take tests in multiple sessions rather than one sitting
- Use of reference materials that reduce frustration (formula sheets, word banks)

- Alternative test formats (multiple choice instead of essay if writing triggers dysregulation)

Social/emotional accommodations support regulation and positive interactions:

- Break card allowing student to take movement breaks without asking permission

- Access to sensory tools (fidget toys, stress balls) during class

- Daily check-in with trusted adult (counselor, behavior specialist, favorite teacher)

- Social skills instruction in small group or individual settings

- Buddy system pairing student with regulated peer for activities

- Modified expectations during known difficult times (after-lunch dysregulation, end of day exhaustion)

Behavioral accommodations address DMDD-specific challenges:

- Behavior intervention plan with clear triggers, preventive strategies, and de-escalation techniques

- Positive behavior support focusing on reinforcing regulation efforts rather than punishing dysregulation

- Time-out procedures that serve as regulation breaks rather than punishment

- Modified consequences recognizing that explosive behavior stems from disability, not willful defiance

- Home-school communication system alerting parents to rough days so they can prepare support

Crisis intervention accommodations prepare for explosive episodes:

- Designated crisis space where student goes during explosions with staff trained to manage crisis

- Safety plan for protecting student, staff, and classmates if severe explosion occurs

- Crisis team that responds when student escalates beyond teacher's ability to manage

- Post-crisis reintegration plan for student's return to classroom after explosion

- Trauma-informed practices protecting other students while supporting struggling student

Case Example: Brandon's Comprehensive Accommodation Plan

Ten-year-old Brandon's IEP included twenty-three separate accommodations addressing his DMDD symptoms. His most effective accommodations included:

Morning check-in: Brandon met with the school counselor for five minutes every morning, rating his mood and stress level. This check-in allowed the counselor to alert Brandon's teacher if Brandon started the day already dysregulated, prompting increased support and reduced demands that day.

Break card system: Brandon kept a laminated card at his desk that he could place on the teacher's desk when he needed a five-minute walk. He didn't need to ask permission or explain. The teacher saw the card and nodded. Brandon walked the school hallways with a predetermined route, returned, and resumed work. This system prevented escalation by allowing Brandon to catch himself early.

Modified math assignments: Math triggered Brandon's most intense frustration. Instead of completing thirty problems, Brandon completed ten problems carefully checked for understanding. Instead of timed tests (which caused immediate dysregulation), Brandon took tests untimed in the learning support room.

Afternoon sensory break: After lunch, Brandon spent fifteen minutes in the occupational therapy sensory room doing heavy work activities (pushing weighted cart, jumping on trampoline, squeezing therapy putty). This break regulated his nervous system before afternoon classes.

Behavior intervention plan: When Brandon showed early escalation signs (heavy sighs, pencil tapping, body tension), his teacher prompted break card use. If Brandon escalated to mid-level (louder voice, minor aggressive language), the teacher sent a pre-arranged text to the counselor who came to walk Brandon to the calm room. If Brandon reached full explosion, the teacher cleared other students from the immediate area, removed dangerous objects, and called the crisis team.

These accommodations didn't eliminate Brandon's DMDD symptoms but made school manageable. His explosions decreased from daily to weekly, then to several times monthly. His academic performance improved as he spent more time learning and less time dysregulated. He developed better awareness of his own regulation state and started using accommodations proactively.

Advocating Without Alienating

Parents of children with DMDD often feel caught between advocating effectively for their child's needs and maintaining positive relationships with school staff. Strong advocacy requires persistence and sometimes pushback, but alienating educators makes collaboration difficult and may ultimately harm your child.

Approach advocacy strategically:

Start collaboratively. Before adversarial tactics, try partnership approaches. Assume good faith—most educators genuinely want to help. Present concerns as opportunities to problem-solve together rather than accusations of failure.

Document everything. Keep records of all communication with school (emails, notes from phone calls, meeting summaries). Document your child's symptoms, incidents at school, and how symptoms affect educational performance. Documentation protects you if relationships deteriorate and legal processes become necessary.

Know your rights. Read and understand IDEA, Section 504, and your state's special education regulations. Organizations like Wrightslaw provide excellent parent advocacy resources. Understanding legal rights allows you to advocate from informed position rather than hoping schools will offer appropriate services voluntarily.

Pick your battles. Not every disagreement requires escalation. Save energy and relationship capital for issues that significantly impact your child's education and well-being. Let minor issues go when possible.

Use the chain of command. Start with teachers and school counselors. If issues aren't resolved, move to special education coordinators or assistant principals. Save principals and district administrators for serious problems that haven't resolved at lower levels.

Request evaluations in writing. Federal law requires schools to respond to written evaluation requests within specific timeframes. Verbal requests don't carry the same weight.

Attend all meetings. IEP and 504 meetings provide formal opportunities to advocate. Prepare for meetings by listing issues to address, bringing supporting documentation, and drafting proposed accommodations or goals.

Bring support. You can bring an advocate, attorney, or supportive friend to meetings. Additional people can take notes, provide emotional support, and strengthen your position.

Stay calm and professional. However angry or frustrated you feel, maintaining composure during meetings serves your child better than emotional outbursts. If you need to say something strongly, practice beforehand and deliver it calmly.

Follow up in writing. After meetings, send emails summarizing agreements, requesting clarification of unclear points, and documenting any disagreements. Written records create paper trails that protect your child.

Escalate when necessary. If schools refuse appropriate services, ignore accommodation plans, or violate legal requirements, escalation becomes necessary. Options include filing complaints with state education departments, requesting mediation, or initiating due process. These processes can be adversarial and damage relationships, but sometimes protecting your child requires it.

Repair relationships when possible. Even after conflict, working relationships matter. When issues resolve, acknowledge school staff efforts and express appreciation. Relationships can recover if both parties value the child's welfare above past disagreements.

Case Example: The Henderson Family's Advocacy Journey

The Henderson family's advocacy for their daughter Zoe illustrates both collaboration and escalation. Zoe's DMDD symptoms worsened in fifth grade, with daily explosions disrupting her class. The school suspended Zoe repeatedly, reaching eight days by November. Her parents requested an IEP evaluation to develop supports preventing suspensions. The school resisted, arguing that Zoe's behavior was willful defiance, not disability-related.

The Hendersons remained calm but firm. They documented Zoe's suspensions, collected letters from her psychiatrist and therapist explaining DMDD, and formally requested evaluation in writing citing IDEA requirements. When the school delayed, they filed a state complaint. The state found the school had violated timelines for responding to evaluation requests and ordered immediate evaluation.

The evaluation qualified Zoe for an IEP under emotional disturbance. During IEP development, the school proposed minimal services—one thirty-minute counseling session monthly. The Hendersons brought their own proposed IEP including daily check-ins, behavior intervention plan, crisis support, and extensive accommodations. Negotiations were tense. The school expressed concern about cost and staff availability. The Hendersons maintained that Zoe needed these services to access education and that cost couldn't be the determining factor.

They reached a compromise—the school agreed to most requested services for a trial period with data collection to evaluate effectiveness. After three months, data showed Zoe's explosions decreased from daily to twice weekly and her academic engagement increased significantly. The services became permanent IEP components.

Throughout this process, the Hendersons tried maintaining positive relationships. They thanked staff members who helped Zoe. They acknowledged the school's resource constraints while insisting on appropriate services. They celebrated successes. When Zoe had a good week, they sent appreciative emails. This balanced approach—firm advocacy with relationship maintenance—helped them achieve necessary services while preserving working relationships for Zoe's remaining years at the school.

School success for children with DMDD requires educational team members understanding the disorder, implementing appropriate accommodations, and maintaining communication and collaboration between home and school. The process often proves frustrating and exhausting, but appropriate educational supports make the difference between a child who feels like a failure and one who accesses learning, develops skills, and works toward their potential despite neurological challenges. This work, combined with treatment, daily life management, and whole-family support, creates the foundation for children with DMDD to grow, heal, and ultimately thrive.

Critical Points for Educational Advocacy

- Teachers and administrators often lack DMDD-specific training, requiring parents to educate while building collaborative partnerships

- Explaining neuroscience helps reframe behavior from willful defiance to neurological challenge requiring support

- Regular communication, shared problem-solving, and acknowledging teacher challenges build goodwill that supports long-term success

- 504 Plans provide accommodations for accessing curriculum; IEPs provide accommodations plus specialized instruction and stronger procedural protections

- Children with DMDD often need IEPs due to requiring specialized instruction beyond simple accommodations

- Effective accommodations address environmental factors, schedule and routine, assignments, testing, social-emotional needs, behavior, and crisis intervention

- Strategic advocacy balances persistence in securing appropriate services with relationship maintenance through professional communication, documentation, and willingness to compromise on non-essential issues

- Escalation to formal processes (complaints, mediation, due process) sometimes becomes necessary to protect educational access despite relationship costs

Chapter 6: Understanding Sibling Impact

Your nine-year-old daughter asks if she can sleep at her friend's house every weekend. Not just sometimes—every single weekend. When you probe gently, she admits the truth: she doesn't feel safe at home. Her brother's explosions terrify her. She never knows when the next one will happen or if this time he might hurt her. She feels guilty for feeling this way because she loves her brother, but the fear is real and constant. This is the reality for siblings of children with DMDD—children who become casualties of a disorder they didn't choose and often don't understand.

The Trauma of Living in a DMDD Household

Siblings of children with DMDD experience their home as a war zone. The comparison is not dramatic exaggeration. Research on siblings of children with severe emotional disturbances shows they display symptoms consistent with trauma exposure— hypervigilance, anxiety, sleep problems, and difficulty feeling safe even in supposedly secure environments.

The trauma comes from multiple sources operating simultaneously. First, siblings witness violence and chaos regularly. They see their brother or sister rage, throw objects, destroy property, and sometimes physically attack family members. They hear screaming that goes on for thirty or forty minutes. They watch their parents struggle to manage explosions, sometimes getting hurt in the process. This repeated exposure to violence affects developing nervous systems, teaching children that their world is fundamentally unsafe.

Second, siblings often become targets. A child with DMDD explodes at whoever happens to be nearby. Siblings might be hit, kicked, or have objects thrown at them. Their belongings get destroyed during rages. Their attempts at normal sibling interaction—asking to play, borrowing something, making an innocent comment—can trigger explosions. Siblings learn to suppress normal childhood behaviors out of fear of provoking their brother or sister.

Third, siblings experience chronic unpredictability. They can't anticipate when explosions will occur or what might trigger them. The child with DMDD might be calm one moment and raging the next. Plans get cancelled. Family outings end abruptly. Normal routines dissolve into crisis management. This unpredictability creates ongoing stress because children can't prepare or protect themselves.

Fourth, siblings lose parental attention and emotional availability. Parents consumed with managing DMDD symptoms have less energy, time, and patience for other children. Siblings notice. They see their parents drop everything when their brother or sister escalates but have no time to help with homework or attend their soccer games. They watch their parents' exhaustion and fear that they're adding to the burden by having normal needs.

Fifth, siblings often feel responsible for managing the home environment. They might try to prevent explosions by monitoring their sibling's mood, avoiding triggers, or keeping younger siblings out of the way. They take on caregiver roles inappropriate for their age, sacrificing their own childhood to maintain fragile household stability.

Case Example: The Wilson Family—Seven-Year-Old Chloe

76

Chloe's brother Jake had DMDD, and his explosions occurred multiple times daily. Chloe developed elaborate strategies for managing her own behavior to minimize Jake's rages. She stopped inviting friends over because Jake's explosions embarrassed her. She gave Jake whatever he wanted—her toys, her snacks, control of the TV—to keep him calm. She became hypervigilant, monitoring Jake constantly for early signs of escalation so she could disappear before explosions started.

Chloe's teacher noticed changes. Chloe seemed anxious and had difficulty concentrating. She startled easily at sudden noises. She spent recess alone rather than playing with other children. When the teacher contacted Chloe's mother about these concerns, the mother broke down crying. She'd been so focused on Jake's treatment that she'd failed to notice how profoundly Jake's DMDD was affecting Chloe.

Chloe's mother arranged for Chloe to see a therapist who specialized in trauma. During play therapy sessions, Chloe revealed her constant fear. She drew pictures of her home as a dark, scary place with monsters. She played out scenarios where the little sister doll hid under the bed while the brother doll raged. She told the therapist she felt safest at school because "Jake isn't there to get mad."

The therapist diagnosed Chloe with anxiety disorder and symptoms of traumatic stress related to chronic exposure to her brother's violence. Treatment included teaching Chloe that she wasn't responsible for preventing Jake's explosions, creating a safety plan for when explosions occurred, and helping Chloe's parents understand that Chloe needed protection and reassurance even though Jake's needs seemed more urgent.

Emotional Burden and Silent Suffering

Many siblings of children with DMDD suffer silently, never expressing the full extent of their emotional burden. They

develop what researchers call "well-child syndrome"—
appearing to function normally or even exceptionally well while
privately struggling with significant distress.

Several factors drive this silent suffering:

Guilt about their feelings prevents siblings from speaking up.
They know their brother or sister has a disorder and can't help
the explosive behavior. They know their parents are
overwhelmed. They feel guilty for resenting their sibling, for
feeling angry about missed activities, for wishing their family
were different. This guilt makes them hide their true feelings,
presenting a facade of understanding and acceptance while
privately hurting.

Fear of adding to parental stress silences siblings. They see
their parents' exhaustion and worry. They don't want to create
more problems by admitting they're struggling. They think,
"Mom and Dad have enough to deal with. I can handle this on
my own." So they suppress their needs and act stronger than
they feel.

Lack of language to describe their experience limits siblings'
ability to ask for help. Young children especially can't articulate
that they feel traumatized, resentful, neglected, or scared. They
know something feels wrong but lack words to explain what
they need.

Minimization by adults teaches siblings that their feelings don't
matter. Adults might say, "Your brother can't help it. You need to
be understanding," or "We all have to make sacrifices for the
family." While adults intend to teach compassion and patience,
siblings hear that their feelings are invalid or selfish. They learn
to hide those feelings rather than expressing them.

Parentification occurs when siblings take on caretaking roles
for their parents or the child with DMDD. They might comfort
their mother after a particularly bad explosion, explain to

relatives why the family can't attend gatherings, or try to cheer up parents who seem sad. This role reversal—children caring for adults—prevents siblings from being cared for themselves.

The emotional burden manifests in various ways. Some siblings develop anxiety disorders, experiencing excessive worry, sleep problems, or physical symptoms like stomachaches and headaches. Others develop depression, showing sad mood, loss of interest in activities, or changes in eating and sleeping. Some become parentified and overly responsible, acting more like mini-adults than children. Others act out behaviorally, getting in trouble at school or home as their only outlet for difficult emotions.

Research shows that siblings of children with severe emotional disturbances are at increased risk for developing their own mental health problems, including anxiety, depression, and behavioral disorders. The chronic stress of living with a sibling's DMDD takes a measurable toll on mental health and development.

Case Example: The Martinez Family—Thirteen-Year-Old Diego

Diego's sister Lucia had DMDD, and Diego spent his adolescent years watching his family revolve around her needs. Diego appeared to handle the situation well. He made good grades, played on the soccer team, and never complained about missed family activities or cancelled plans. His parents praised him for being "the easy one" and "so understanding about Lucia's condition."

Privately, Diego was falling apart. He felt angry constantly but couldn't express it. He resented Lucia for dominating the family. He resented his parents for never having time for him. He felt guilty for these feelings because he knew Lucia had a real disorder. The combination of anger and guilt created internal conflict that Diego couldn't resolve.

Diego began self-medicating with marijuana at age fourteen. Getting high provided temporary relief from the constant tension he felt. His parents, distracted by Lucia's treatment, didn't notice. By fifteen, Diego was using daily and his grades started dropping. A teacher who noticed changes contacted Diego's parents, expressing concern about possible substance use.

Diego's parents were shocked. Diego had seemed fine. How had they missed this? In family therapy, Diego finally expressed what he'd been holding inside for years: "I don't matter in this family. Everything is about Lucia. Nobody cares if I'm okay or not. I just have to be perfect and not cause any problems while my sister destroys everything."

This revelation devastated Diego's parents but also opened the door to healing. They recognized that Diego's substance use was a desperate attempt to cope with feelings he couldn't express safely. Treatment addressed both Diego's substance use and the underlying family issues that contributed to it. Diego needed space to express his anger and resentment without judgment, reassurance that his needs mattered, and individual attention from his parents.

Age-Specific Impacts on Different Developmental Stages

The effects of living with a sibling who has DMDD vary by the sibling's age and developmental stage. Younger children, older children, and teenagers experience and interpret their sibling's condition differently.

Young children (ages 3-7) have limited understanding of DMDD as a disorder. They know their sibling gets very angry and scary but can't grasp that this stems from neurological differences rather than choice. Young children often blame themselves, thinking they cause their sibling's explosions by being bad or annoying. They might believe they could prevent explosions if they were better behaved.

Young siblings often develop separation anxiety, becoming clingy and fearful when parents leave. They might regress developmentally—returning to bedwetting after being potty-trained, wanting bottles after being weaned, or using baby talk. They have nightmares about their sibling or scary monsters that represent the sibling's rage. They might show aggressive behavior at school or daycare, mimicking the violence they witness at home.

Young children need concrete reassurance that they're safe, that the explosions aren't their fault, and that parents will protect them. They need simple explanations of their sibling's condition at their comprehension level. They need maintained routines to provide stability amidst chaos.

School-age children (ages 8-12) develop more sophisticated understanding of DMDD as a medical condition but still struggle with the emotional impact. They understand intellectually that their sibling can't always control the behavior but feel angry and resentful anyway. This creates cognitive dissonance—their thoughts and feelings don't match.

School-age siblings often experience social isolation. They stop inviting friends over out of fear their sibling will explode and embarrass them. They decline invitations to friends' houses because they feel guilty having fun while their family struggles. They might be bullied at school if peers know about their sibling's behavior problems.

These children frequently become parentified, taking on caregiving roles for younger siblings or even for the child with DMDD. They might monitor their sibling's mood, try to prevent explosions, or attempt to de-escalate situations. They sacrifice their own childhood to help maintain family functioning.

School-age siblings need help understanding that DMDD is a real condition but that their feelings about it are still valid. They need permission to feel angry, sad, or resentful even though their sibling has a disorder. They need individual time with parents and opportunities to pursue their own interests without guilt.

Teenagers (ages 13-18) face unique challenges related to their developmental need for independence and identity formation. Teenagers naturally begin separating from family and spending more time with peers. But teenagers with siblings who have DMDD often feel trapped between normal developmental needs and family obligations.

Adolescent siblings might feel angry that their family situation interferes with normal teenage experiences—dating, driving, hanging out with friends, participating in activities. They might feel ashamed of their family and hide their home situation from peers. They might rush toward independence prematurely, moving out at eighteen or spending all their time away from home to escape the chaos.

Teenagers also worry about the future—will they be expected to care for their sibling as adults? What if they want to move away for college but their parents need help? How will their sibling's condition affect their own life choices? These concerns add stress during an already challenging developmental period.

Some teenagers respond by becoming overachievers, pouring energy into academics, athletics, or other pursuits where they can excel and receive recognition. Others act out through substance use, risky behavior, or defiance. Still others withdraw, becoming depressed and isolated.

Teenagers need acknowledgment that their developmental needs for independence are legitimate and important. They need explicit permission to build lives separate from their sibling's disorder. They need honest conversations about future expectations and reassurance that they're not solely responsible for their sibling's lifetime care.

Case Example: The Thompson Family—Three Siblings at Different Ages

The Thompson family had three children: five-year-old Emma, ten-year-old Caleb, and sixteen-year-old Sophia. Their middle child, Caleb, had DMDD. His explosions affected his sisters differently based on their ages.

Emma, at five, showed the most obvious trauma symptoms. She had frequent nightmares and refused to sleep in her own room. She needed her mother present constantly and cried when dropped off at kindergarten. She became aggressive with peers, hitting and pushing when frustrated. Emma couldn't articulate her fear, but her behavior screamed distress.

Sophia, at sixteen, dealt with the situation by avoiding home. She took every opportunity to be elsewhere—staying late after school for activities, spending weekends at friends' houses, working part-time. When forced to be home, Sophia stayed in her room with headphones on. She'd become an excellent student and athlete partly because achievement provided escape and recognition. But Sophia also felt tremendous guilt about wanting to leave for college, knowing her departure would leave her parents with less support.

The family entered therapy after Emma's kindergarten teacher expressed serious concerns about Emma's behavior and emotional state. During family sessions, each child's different needs became clear. Emma needed immediate trauma intervention, safety planning, and lots of reassurance. Caleb needed continued DMDD treatment plus help understanding how his condition affected his sisters. Sophia needed permission to pursue independence without guilt and explicit conversations about future expectations.

The therapist helped the parents see that all three children needed individual attention and support, not just Caleb. Emma started play therapy. Sophia had individual sessions to process her feelings and plan for college without guilt. The parents learned to make time for each child separately, even fifteen minutes of individual attention made differences. The family developed a safety plan for Emma during Caleb's explosions, including a safe space Emma could go and a signal she could use to alert her parents she needed comfort afterward.

Siblings of children with DMDD pay a high price for a disorder they didn't cause and can't control. Recognizing their trauma, acknowledging their silent suffering, and addressing their age-specific needs are not optional extras in DMDD treatment—they're necessary components of family healing. The next chapter addresses what siblings need to survive and, eventually, thrive despite the challenges their family faces.

What Siblings Need You to Know

- Siblings experience genuine trauma from repeated exposure to violence, chaos, and unpredictability in DMDD households

- Multiple trauma sources affect siblings simultaneously including witnessing violence, becoming targets, experiencing unpredictability, losing parental attention, and feeling responsible for household management

- Many siblings suffer silently due to guilt, fear of adding to parental stress, lack of language to describe experiences, adult minimization of their feelings, and parentification

- Silent suffering manifests as anxiety disorders, depression, parentification, behavioral problems, or substance use in older siblings

- Age affects how siblings experience DMDD—young children blame themselves and show regression, school-age children struggle with cognitive dissonance and social isolation, and teenagers feel trapped between developmental needs and family obligations

- All siblings need recognition of their trauma, validation of their feelings, age-appropriate support, and explicit permission to have their own needs and lives separate from their sibling's disorder

Chapter 7: Supporting Siblings

The pediatrician's office called about your daughter's physical exam. Everything checked out fine medically, but your daughter told the nurse she wished she had a disorder like her brother because then maybe you'd pay attention to her. The comment stopped your heart. You've been so focused on managing your son's DMDD that you missed your daughter's desperate bid for recognition. She doesn't actually want a disorder—she wants you to notice she exists, she matters, and she needs you too. This realization marks the beginning of actively supporting the forgotten children in families affected by DMDD.

Six Essential Things Siblings Need

Research and clinical experience with siblings of children who have severe emotional disturbances reveal six non-negotiable needs that these children must have met to survive the experience without lasting harm.

1. Information and Understanding

Siblings need age-appropriate information about DMDD—what it is, what causes it, how it affects their brother or sister, and why treatment takes time. Without information, siblings create their own explanations, usually involving self-blame or misunderstanding.

Young children need simple explanations: "Your brother's brain works differently. He feels frustration much bigger than other people, and he hasn't learned how to calm those big feelings yet.

That's not your fault, and it's not his fault—it's just how his brain works right now. We're helping him learn better ways to handle frustration."

School-age children can understand more details: "Your sister has a condition called DMDD. It means her brain has trouble regulating emotions. Things that might annoy you a little bit feel huge to her. She's not choosing to explode—her nervous system reacts too strongly, too fast. She's working with a therapist to develop better control, but it takes a long time to change how brains work."

Teenagers benefit from full information including neurobiological explanations, treatment approaches, and honest discussion of prognosis. They can handle knowing that DMDD is serious, treatment is difficult, and outcomes are uncertain. They often appreciate being treated as mature enough to understand the full picture.

Information alone isn't enough—siblings also need space to ask questions and express doubts. Create regular opportunities for siblings to ask anything without judgment. Some questions might be difficult: "Will my brother ever get better?" "Why can't the doctors fix this?" "Is this genetic—will my kids have it?" Answer honestly while providing reassurance where possible.

2. Validation of Their Feelings

Siblings need explicit permission to have negative feelings about their sibling and their situation. They need adults to say, "It's okay to feel angry. It's okay to wish your family were different. Those feelings don't make you a bad person."

Many siblings believe that having negative feelings about a sibling with a disorder makes them horrible people. They think they should be more understanding, more patient, more compassionate. Adults often reinforce this message, saying things like "Your sister can't help it—you need to be more understanding." While technically true, this message invalidates the sibling's legitimate feelings of frustration, anger, fear, and resentment.

Validate specific feelings: "I know you're angry that we had to leave your game early because of your brother's meltdown. That's completely understandable. You practiced hard and wanted to finish the game." Validation doesn't solve the problem, but it helps siblings feel seen and understood.

Siblings also need validation that their needs matter even though their sibling's needs seem more urgent. Say explicitly: "Your brother's needs are urgent right now, but that doesn't mean your needs aren't important. You matter just as much as he does. Sometimes we have to handle his crisis first, but we'll always come back to make sure you're okay too."

3. Safety Assurances

Siblings need concrete assurance that adults will keep them safe. This includes physical safety during explosions and emotional safety in the household overall.

Develop a safety plan specifically for siblings:

- Identify a safe space siblings can go during explosions (their room with a lock, a neighbor's house, a specific room away from the crisis)

- Create a signal siblings can use to alert adults they feel unsafe (a hand signal, a code word, texting a specific emoji)

- Establish clear rules about physical boundaries (the child with DMDD may not enter the sibling's room during escalation, certain objects must be secured so they can't be thrown)

- Practice the safety plan during calm times so siblings know exactly what to do

If the child with DMDD has hurt siblings physically, take this seriously. Consider interventions like installing locks on bedroom doors, separating children during high-risk times, or even temporary living arrangements if violence is severe and uncontrolled. Siblings cannot heal from trauma if they remain in ongoing danger.

Beyond physical safety, siblings need emotional safety to express their feelings, ask questions, and have needs without fear of repercussion or judgment. Create specific times when siblings can talk privately about how they're feeling without the child with DMDD present.

4. Individual Time and Attention

Siblings desperately need one-on-one time with parents where they receive full attention without interruption or distraction. This doesn't require expensive outings or elaborate plans—fifteen minutes of undivided attention makes a difference.

Schedule individual time regularly (weekly is ideal) and treat it as sacred. Don't cancel for anything short of genuine emergency. During this time, put phones away, don't discuss the child with DMDD, and focus entirely on the sibling. Do whatever the sibling wants within reason—play a game, take a walk, bake cookies, just talk.

Some siblings need more time than others. Younger children might need daily check-ins plus weekly special time. Teenagers might want less frequent but longer periods of individual attention. Ask siblings what would feel meaningful to them.

Both parents need to spend individual time with siblings when possible. If one parent becomes the primary DMDD crisis manager while the other parent focuses on siblings, this can work, but ideally both parents maintain connection with all children.

Individual attention communicates powerful messages: You matter. I see you. Your needs are important. I care about your life beyond how it relates to your sibling. You're valued for who you are, not just for being understanding about your sibling's condition.

5. Opportunities for Normal Childhood

Siblings need permission and support to pursue normal childhood activities without guilt. They need to attend their soccer games, birthday parties, and school events without worrying about their family situation. They need time with friends. They need to be kids.

Many siblings restrict their own lives because they feel guilty having fun while their family struggles. They decline invitations, quit activities they enjoy, and isolate themselves. Parents need to actively counter this by encouraging siblings to maintain normal activities.

Sometimes logistics require creative problem-solving. If one parent must stay home to manage the child with DMDD, the other parent can take siblings to activities. Extended family, neighbors, or friends can transport siblings when both parents are needed at home. Some families arrange for respite care providers to supervise the child with DMDD so parents can attend siblings' events.

Normalize talking about the sibling's life outside the family. Ask about friends, school, interests, and activities with genuine curiosity. Celebrate their achievements even when those achievements seem small compared to the ongoing crisis of managing DMDD.

Siblings also need space to make their own choices about how much they want to be involved in their sibling's treatment and care. Some siblings want to attend therapy sessions or participate in family meetings. Others need separation and shouldn't be forced to participate beyond what feels comfortable.

6. Their Own Support System

Siblings benefit from support systems separate from the family that provide additional outlets for processing their experience. This might include therapy, support groups, school counseling, or relationships with trusted adults who understand their situation.

Individual therapy helps siblings process trauma, develop coping skills, and work through difficult feelings in a safe environment. A therapist serves as the sibling's advocate, keeping the sibling's needs central without having to balance them against the child with DMDD's needs.

Sibling support groups connect children with others facing similar situations. Knowing they're not alone reduces isolation and shame. Groups provide peer support and normalize the experience of having a sibling with severe behavioral issues.

Some siblings benefit from mentoring relationships with adults outside the immediate family—teachers, coaches, relatives, or family friends who can provide additional attention and support. These adults offer perspective, encouragement, and sometimes practical help like transportation to activities or a quiet place to study.

School counselors can provide check-ins, support during difficult days, and advocacy if the sibling's academic performance suffers due to home stress. Inform key school staff about the family situation so they can watch for signs the sibling is struggling and offer appropriate support.

Case Example: The Roberts Family Implements All Six Needs

After their son Tyler was diagnosed with DMDD, the Roberts family realized their daughter Maya, age nine, was showing signs of significant distress. Maya had become withdrawn, her grades dropped, and she told her teacher she hated her family. The teacher referred the family to counseling.

The family therapist helped the Roberts develop a plan addressing all six of Maya's needs:

Information: Maya's parents sat down with her and explained DMDD in detail. They used a book about brain differences to help Maya understand. They encouraged questions and revisited the conversation multiple times as Maya processed the information.

Validation: Maya's mother started saying things like, "I know you feel angry when Tyler's explosions ruin our plans. That anger makes sense. I feel frustrated too." This validation helped Maya feel less guilty about her negative feelings.

Safety: They created a safety plan. During Tyler's explosions, Maya went to her room (they installed a lock), put on headphones, and listened to music. Afterward, one parent always checked on Maya, asked how she was feeling, and offered comfort.

Individual time: Each parent committed to one hour weekly alone with Maya. Her father took Maya to breakfast every Saturday morning. Her mother and Maya had "girls' night" every Friday with movies and manicures. During these times, they didn't discuss Tyler unless Maya brought him up.

Normal activities: Maya loved gymnastics but had quit because Tyler's behaviors often prevented her parents from attending her classes and meets. They arranged for Maya's grandmother to take her to gymnastics and attend her meets when they couldn't. This allowed Maya to continue something she loved without guilt.

Support system: Maya started seeing a therapist weekly. The therapist helped Maya process her feelings about Tyler and develop coping strategies. Maya also joined a sibling support group where she met other kids with siblings who had behavioral disorders.

Within six months, Maya's mood improved significantly. Her grades returned to normal. She reported feeling less anxious and angry. Most telling, Maya told her therapist, "I still don't like Tyler's explosions, but I don't feel invisible anymore. My parents see me now."

Creating Safety and Predictability

Beyond the six essential needs, siblings require specific environmental modifications that increase their sense of safety and predictability in an otherwise chaotic household.

Physical safety measures protect siblings during explosions:

- Secure dangerous objects that might be thrown or used as weapons
- Create barriers preventing the child with DMDD from accessing siblings' rooms during escalation
- Establish no-hit zones where the child with DMDD isn't allowed during peak dysregulation times
- Teach siblings how to protect themselves if attacked (blocking, moving away, calling for help)
- Install locks on bedroom doors so siblings can create secure space

Predictable routines provide stability amidst unpredictability:

- Maintain consistent meal times, bedtimes, and morning routines as much as possible

- Preserve rituals that matter to siblings (bedtime stories, weekend pancakes, game nights)

- Create backup plans for when DMDD symptoms disrupt primary plans

- Use visual schedules showing what to expect each day

- Communicate changes as far in advance as possible

Designated safe spaces give siblings retreat options:

- Identify rooms where siblings can go during explosions that are truly safe (the child with DMDD won't follow)

- Stock safe spaces with comforting items (stuffed animals, books, art supplies, sensory tools)

- Ensure siblings have access to these spaces whenever needed without asking permission

- Teach siblings they're not abandoning the family by protecting themselves

Communication protocols help siblings know what's happening:

- Develop simple signals parents can use to indicate situation severity (thumbs up means everything's okay, flat hand means stay in room, etc.)

- Text or call siblings if DMDD crisis occurs while they're away from home so they know what to expect when returning

- Debrief after significant explosions, checking how siblings are feeling and what they need

- Create family meetings where everyone can share concerns and problem-solve together

Preservation of special events communicates that siblings' milestones matter:

- Attend siblings' important events (recitals, games, performances) even if it requires arranging alternative care for the child with DMDD

- Celebrate siblings' birthdays fully without letting DMDD symptoms overshadow their special day

- Take siblings on occasional outings without the child with DMDD so they experience family time without explosions

- Document siblings' achievements with the same attention given to the child with DMDD's treatment progress

Case Example: The Kim Family's Safety and Predictability Systems

The Kim family had two daughters—eight-year-old Jenna with DMDD and eleven-year-old Rachel. Rachel had become increasingly anxious and fearful at home after several incidents where Jenna physically attacked her during explosions.

The family worked with their therapist to create multiple systems addressing safety and predictability:

They installed a lock on Rachel's bedroom door. Rachel kept the key and could lock herself in anytime she felt unsafe. The parents promised they'd never ask Rachel to unlock the door during one of Jenna's explosions—that space was completely Rachel's.

They created a color-coded system for communicating household mood. A green paper plate on the kitchen bulletin board meant everything was calm. Yellow meant someone was having a hard day and everyone should be extra patient. Red meant active crisis and Rachel should go to her safe space. This visual system helped Rachel assess safety without asking questions that might trigger Jenna.

They maintained sacred routines for Rachel. Sunday evenings were always game night with Rachel. Even if Jenna had multiple explosions that day, they played games with Rachel while Jenna watched TV in another room or a babysitter stayed with Jenna. Rachel's Tuesday afternoon art class continued no matter what. Her mother or a carpool arrangement ensured Rachel never missed class due to Jenna's symptoms.

They developed a crisis communication plan. If Rachel was at a friend's house and a major explosion occurred at home, her parents would text her a predetermined emoji. This alerted Rachel that home was in crisis mode, and she could make the choice to stay at her friend's longer if needed.

These systems transformed Rachel's experience. She reported feeling safer knowing she could protect herself, less anxious because she could assess home safety before entering, and more valued because her needs were prioritized through maintained routines despite her sister's condition.

Individual Time and Validation

While listed as one of the six essential needs, individual time and validation deserve expanded discussion because they're both critically important and commonly neglected.

Individual time requires intentionality. It doesn't happen accidentally. Parents must schedule it, protect it, and treat it as seriously as medical appointments. The time doesn't need to be lengthy—quality matters more than quantity—but it needs to be regular and uninterrupted.

During individual time:

- Put away all phones and eliminate all distractions

- Follow the sibling's lead about activities and conversation topics

- Don't discuss the child with DMDD unless the sibling initiates

- Show genuine interest in the sibling's life, feelings, thoughts, and experiences

- Provide physical affection appropriate to the child's age and preferences

- Make the sibling feel like the most important person in your world for that moment

Some parents resist individual time because they feel guilty. If they're spending time with the sibling, who's managing the child with DMDD? How can they have fun when their family is in crisis? This guilt must be overcome. Individual time with siblings isn't selfish or optional—it's necessary preventive intervention protecting siblings' mental health.

Validation goes beyond saying "I understand." Real validation communicates that the sibling's feelings make sense given their circumstances, that those feelings are acceptable, and that the sibling doesn't need to hide or change legitimate emotions.

Validation includes:

- Naming feelings accurately: "You seem angry about missing the party"

- Acknowledging feelings without minimizing: "That is disappointing" not "It's not a big deal"

- Connecting feelings to circumstances: "Of course you feel frustrated—you've been looking forward to this all week"

- Separating feelings from actions: "It's okay to feel angry; it's not okay to hit"

- Avoiding the word "but": Don't say "I know you're upset BUT your brother can't help it" because "but" negates everything before it

Validation doesn't solve problems but it helps siblings feel understood. Feeling understood reduces emotional distress even when circumstances can't change immediately.

Case Example: The Anderson Family—Validation Transforms Cameron

Twelve-year-old Cameron had a younger brother with DMDD. For years, Cameron suppressed his feelings, insisting he was fine when clearly he wasn't. His parents praised him for being "so mature" and "so understanding," never realizing this praise reinforced Cameron's pattern of denying his true feelings.

Cameron's mask cracked when he punched a hole in his bedroom wall after his parents missed his award ceremony to handle another DMDD crisis with his brother. This outburst, so unlike Cameron's usual controlled behavior, alarmed his parents. They sought help.

The family therapist taught Cameron's parents proper validation. They started saying things like:

- "You worked hard on that project. Missing your ceremony was a real loss"

- "I'd be angry too if I had to give up something important because of someone else's problem"

- "Your feelings about your brother are complicated—you love him and resent him at the same time. That's normal given what you live with"

Cameron initially resisted this validation. He'd built an identity around being the good child, the one who didn't need attention. Accepting validation felt uncomfortable, almost threatening. But gradually, Cameron began opening up.

He admitted he often felt invisible. He revealed that he sometimes hated his brother and felt terrible about that hatred. He confessed he'd been having thoughts about running away because he couldn't take the chaos anymore.

These admissions led to real help. Cameron started therapy. His parents made concrete changes, including hiring a respite care provider so they could attend Cameron's events. They scheduled weekly individual time with Cameron. Most importantly, they consistently validated Cameron's feelings instead of praising him for suppressing them.

Six months into treatment, Cameron's mother asked how he was doing. Cameron's answer revealed the transformation: "I still hate the situation. I still wish our family were normal. But I don't feel like I have to pretend anymore. You guys actually care how I feel now, not just how well I'm handling it."

Therapy and Support for Siblings

Professional support for siblings isn't a luxury—it's a necessity given the trauma exposure and emotional burden these children carry.

Individual therapy provides siblings with their own advocate and safe space to process complex feelings. Therapists help siblings:

- Understand their sibling's condition without feeling responsible for it

- Process trauma from witnessing violence and chaos

- Develop healthy coping strategies for managing stress

- Challenge distorted beliefs (like self-blame for explosions)

- Express feelings they can't share with parents

- Build self-esteem separate from family chaos

- Develop boundaries protecting their emotional wellbeing

- Plan for their future without excessive guilt about leaving

Therapy modalities particularly helpful for siblings include trauma-focused cognitive behavioral therapy (TF-CBT) for those showing trauma symptoms, play therapy for younger children who can't verbalize their experiences, and cognitive behavioral therapy for older children and teens dealing with anxiety or depression.

Family therapy helps the entire family system adjust to include support for siblings alongside DMDD treatment. Family therapy addresses:

- Communication patterns that exclude or silence siblings

- Redistributing parental attention more equally

- Processing how DMDD affects each family member

- Developing family problem-solving approaches

- Creating safety plans that protect everyone

- Strengthening sibling relationships despite the challenges

Family therapy works best when the therapist explicitly advocates for siblings' needs, not allowing those needs to be overshadowed by the child with DMDD's more obvious and urgent symptoms.

Sibling support groups connect children facing similar situations. These groups typically meet weekly or biweekly and include structured activities helping siblings:

- Share their experiences in a judgment-free environment
- Realize they're not alone in their struggles
- Learn from others' coping strategies
- Receive validation from peers who truly understand
- Practice skills for managing difficult emotions
- Build friendships with others who "get it"

Support groups are particularly valuable for older children and teenagers who may be more comfortable sharing with peers than adults. Groups reduce the isolation many siblings feel.

School-based support can supplement other interventions. School counselors provide:

- Brief check-ins during the school day
- Crisis support when siblings are having particularly hard days
- Academic accommodations if home stress affects school performance
- Social skills groups if siblings struggle with peer relationships
- Liaison services coordinating with outside therapists and family

Inform key school personnel (teachers, counselor, nurse) about the family situation so they can monitor the sibling and offer support proactively rather than waiting for obvious crisis.

Peer relationships provide additional support through friendships with children who may or may not know about the family situation. Some siblings prefer keeping their home life private from friends. Others find it helpful to have trusted friends who know and understand. Support siblings in whichever approach feels comfortable for them.

Encourage siblings to maintain friendships and social connections even when they feel like withdrawing. Social isolation worsens mental health, while social connection protects against stress effects.

Case Example: The Torres Family—Comprehensive Support for Olivia

Nine-year-old Olivia's brother Marcus had severe DMDD with multiple daily explosions. By third grade, Olivia showed signs of trauma including nightmares, school avoidance, stomachaches, and excessive worry. Her parents recognized Olivia needed help beyond what they could provide at home.

Olivia started individual play therapy with a trauma-specialist therapist. During sessions, Olivia drew pictures of scary monsters representing Marcus's rage. She built safe spaces with blocks. She played out scenarios where the little girl figure protected herself during the brother figure's rampage. The therapist taught Olivia that her fear made sense, that Marcus's explosions weren't her fault, and that she could learn to feel safer.

The family attended family therapy biweekly. During these sessions, Olivia practiced expressing her feelings directly. At first, she could only say "I'm fine" when asked how she felt. With the therapist's support and her parents' encouragement,

Olivia eventually said things like "I'm scared when Marcus yells" and "I feel sad that we never do fun stuff as a family."

Olivia joined a sibling support group at a local children's hospital. Six children with siblings who had various behavioral and mental health disorders met weekly for two hours. They did art projects, played games, and talked about their experiences. Olivia formed friendships with two other girls in the group. For the first time, Olivia felt understood by peers.

Her parents informed her teacher and school counselor about the family situation. The counselor started checking in with Olivia twice weekly, asking how things were at home and how Olivia was managing. When Olivia had particularly hard days, the counselor let her spend time in the office doing calming activities.

This comprehensive support network transformed Olivia's functioning. Her nightmares decreased. Her stomachaches resolved. She started smiling again and engaging with classmates. Most importantly, Olivia developed confidence that she could survive her family's challenges without being destroyed by them.

Supporting siblings of children with DMDD requires intentional effort, resources, and commitment. But this investment pays off. Siblings who receive proper support during childhood emerge from the experience resilient rather than traumatized, capable of healthy relationships, and able to pursue their own lives without excessive guilt or lasting damage. The next chapter shifts focus from siblings to the parent partnership, examining how DMDD affects marriages and what couples can do to preserve their relationship while managing this challenging condition.

Essential Support Strategies Siblings Must Receive

- Six non-negotiable needs must be met including information and understanding, validation of feelings, safety assurances, individual time and attention, opportunities for normal childhood, and their own support systems

- Safety measures require both physical protection during explosions and emotional safety to express feelings without judgment

- Predictability comes through maintained routines, backup plans, communication protocols, and preservation of siblings' special events

- Individual time must be scheduled, protected, and treated as sacred, not optional, with full parental attention and no discussion of the child with DMDD

- Validation requires naming feelings accurately, acknowledging them without minimizing, connecting feelings to circumstances, and avoiding words like "but" that negate everything before them

- Professional support including individual therapy, family therapy, sibling support groups, and school-based services provides necessary intervention preventing lasting trauma

- Comprehensive support transforms siblings from traumatized casualties to resilient survivors who can pursue healthy, independent lives

Chapter 8: The Parent Partnership

You haven't had a conversation with your spouse that wasn't about your son's DMDD in three months. You can't recall the last time you laughed together or held hands. You sleep in separate rooms because one of you needs to be alert in case your son explodes in the middle of the night. You argue constantly about everything—discipline approaches, medication decisions, therapy choices, whether to accept the school's latest suspension. You look at your spouse and barely recognize the person you married. DMDD doesn't just affect the child who has it—it affects every relationship in the family, and marriages often bear the heaviest burden.

How DMDD Strains Marriages

Research on parents of children with severe emotional and behavioral disorders shows significantly higher rates of marital conflict, reduced marital satisfaction, and increased divorce risk compared to parents of typically developing children. DMDD creates multiple stressors that systematically damage marital relationships.

Chronic stress depletes the emotional resources couples need to maintain healthy relationships. Managing daily explosions, navigating treatment systems, handling school crises, and coping with your child's suffering creates relentless stress. This stress activates fight-or-flight physiology, making partners more reactive, defensive, and irritable with each other. You snap at your spouse over minor annoyances because your nervous system stays perpetually activated by the major threat of your child's condition.

Exhaustion makes connection nearly impossible. After managing DMDD symptoms all day, parents have nothing left for each other. Emotional exhaustion prevents empathy. Physical exhaustion eliminates any thought of intimacy. Mental exhaustion makes even basic conversation feel overwhelming. You fall into bed at night too tired to talk, too depleted to connect, barely able to manage the necessities before sleep finally comes.

Different coping styles create conflict. One parent might cope through action—researching treatment options, scheduling appointments, implementing behavior plans. The other might need processing time—talking through emotions, grieving losses, questioning decisions. These different styles can feel like judgment or criticism. The research-focused parent sees the processing parent as dwelling on problems instead of solving them. The processing parent sees the research-focused parent as avoiding emotional reality through manic activity.

Disagreement about treatment approaches creates ongoing friction. Should you try medication or exhaust behavioral interventions first? Is this therapist the right fit or should you seek someone else? Should you accept the school's 504 plan or push for an IEP? Should you implement stricter discipline or more permissive approaches? Couples argue about these decisions constantly, each convinced their approach is right and their spouse's is wrong.

Blame and resentment poison relationships. In desperate attempts to understand why your child has DMDD, parents sometimes blame each other. Maybe it's genetic from his family. Maybe it's because she was too permissive when he was younger. Maybe the trauma of that difficult birth caused it.

These blame narratives, even when unspoken, create resentment that damages connection.

Resentment also builds when partners feel they carry unequal loads. One parent becomes the primary crisis manager while the other maintains income. One stays up all night during insomnia episodes while the other sleeps. One handles medical appointments while the other deals with school. Even when division of labor makes practical sense, resentment develops: "You get to go to work and interact with adults while I'm home managing explosions all day." "You get to leave when things get hard while I handle everything."

Loss of shared identity separates couples who once functioned as a team. Before DMDD dominated family life, you were partners with shared interests, goals, and experiences. Now you're co-managers of a crisis, functioning more like coworkers than spouses. You've forgotten what you used to talk about besides your child's symptoms. You can't remember the last time you did something fun together. Your identity as a couple has been consumed by your identity as parents of a child with DMDD.

Lack of time alone prevents relationship maintenance. Date nights feel impossible when finding childcare for a child with DMDD is nearly impossible. Who can you trust to manage explosive behavior? What if there's a crisis while you're gone? How can you relax knowing you'll return to chaos? Many couples abandon attempts at couple time, resigning themselves to functioning as crisis management partners rather than romantic partners.

Sexual intimacy becomes distant memory. Exhaustion kills libido. Stress makes bodies feel unsafe and unable to relax into pleasure. Chronic tension creates physical and emotional distance. Resentment prevents vulnerability. Sleep deprivation makes any use of free time for sleep feel more important than sex. Years might pass with minimal physical intimacy, creating another layer of disconnection.

Grief differences cause misunderstanding. Both parents grieve the child they expected to have and the family life they imagined. But people grieve differently and on different timelines. One parent might still be in denial or bargaining while the other has moved to acceptance. One might need to talk about the grief repeatedly while the other prefers distraction. These differences can feel like lack of support or invalidation.

Case Example: The Miller Marriage in Crisis

Sarah and David Miller had been married twelve years when their son Luke was diagnosed with DMDD. The diagnosis brought relief initially—finally they understood what was wrong. But within a year, their marriage was falling apart.

Sarah handled most of Luke's daily care, including managing explosions, coordinating treatment, and communicating with school. David worked long hours partially out of necessity (they needed income and insurance) and partially out of escape (work was easier than home). Sarah resented David's absence. David resented Sarah's constant reports of Luke's latest crisis.

They disagreed about medication. Sarah wanted to try medications to reduce Luke's suffering and improve family functioning. David worried about side effects and wanted to exhaust behavioral approaches first. They argued about this decision for months, each feeling the other didn't understand or respect their perspective.

They hadn't had sex in eight months. They slept in separate rooms because Luke often woke during the night requiring intervention. They hadn't had a date in over a year. They barely spoke about anything except Luke's treatment, school problems, and logistics.

Sarah finally told David she couldn't continue. She wasn't threatening divorce, but she was admitting the marriage was dying and she didn't know how to save it while also managing Luke's DMDD.

Unified Parenting Approaches

While DMDD strains marriages, developing unified parenting approaches can protect relationships and improve outcomes for the child with DMDD. Unity doesn't mean identical—it means coordinated, respectful, and consistent.

Agree on core principles even when disagreeing on specifics. Core principles might include:

- We're on the same team working toward shared goals

- Our child's DMDD is not our fault or their fault

- We'll make major decisions together, not unilaterally

- We'll present a united front to our child even when we disagree privately

- We'll assume good intentions even when we disagree with execution

These principles provide foundation when specific disagreements arise. You might disagree about whether to try a new medication, but you both want your child to suffer less and function better. Starting from shared goals makes negotiating specific differences easier.

Develop decision-making processes for major choices rather than arguing each decision separately. One effective approach:

1. Research independently: Each parent gathers information from reputable sources about the decision

2. Share findings: Each parent presents what they learned without judgment

3. Express concerns: Each parent states their concerns about different options

4. Identify values: Each parent explains which values (safety, quality of life, financial responsibility) are driving their preferences

5. Compromise or defer: Either find middle ground or agree that one parent's concerns are more pressing for this particular decision with the understanding that next time, it might go differently

6. Support implementation: Whichever approach gets chosen, both parents support it fully and evaluate results together

This process reduces conflicts born from feeling unheard or steamrolled. Both parents contribute, both are heard, and decisions result from discussion rather than argument.

Divide responsibilities based on strengths rather than assuming equal involvement in everything. Maybe one parent handles medical appointments and insurance while the other manages school communication. Maybe one does morning routine while the other handles evenings. Maybe one specializes in prevention strategies while the other manages active crises.

Division of labor works when both partners value all roles equally. The parent who handles day-to-day crises isn't more important than the parent who maintains income and insurance. The parent who attends all therapy appointments isn't working harder than the parent who manages other children's needs. Both roles matter.

Create regular communication routines for discussing DMDD-related issues so they don't dominate all couple interaction. Schedule weekly meetings specifically for this purpose. During the meeting, review the past week, discuss upcoming appointments or decisions, problem-solve current challenges, and plan the next week. Time-limiting these discussions (thirty to sixty minutes) prevents them from consuming your entire relationship.

Outside these scheduled times, try to minimize DMDD-focused conversation. Talk about other topics. Talk about your relationship. Talk about anything except your child's condition. This creates mental space for connection beyond crisis management.

Present unified responses to your child even when you disagree. Children with DMDD, like all children, detect and exploit parental disagreement. If parents respond inconsistently—one permissive, one strict—the child learns to manipulate those differences. Worse, inconsistency worsens the child's dysregulation because predictability reduces anxiety.

If you disagree about how to handle a situation, discuss privately and then present a unified response. If you can't agree immediately, default to one parent's approach temporarily with agreement to revisit. Don't undermine each other in front of the child.

Support your partner's approach even if it's not your preferred method, unless that approach is genuinely harmful. If your spouse implements a strategy you think won't work, let them try it and evaluate results together. Say supportive things: "Your dad has a plan for managing homework time. Let's see how it works." This support strengthens your partnership and models teamwork for your child.

Case Example: The Rodriguez Family Creates Unity

Maria and Carlos Rodriguez had nearly separated over disagreements about their daughter Anna's DMDD treatment. After attending a parenting workshop focused on maintaining marriages during childhood illness, they implemented several strategies.

They established weekly "business meetings" every Sunday evening after Anna went to bed. During these meetings, they reviewed Anna's week, discussed upcoming appointments, made decisions about treatment, and planned logistics. They set a timer for forty-five minutes. When the timer went off, DMDD discussion ended even if they hadn't covered everything.

They divided responsibilities based on their strengths. Maria was organized and detail-oriented, so she managed Anna's medication schedule, tracked behavior data, and coordinated with providers. Carlos was calm during crises, so he became the primary responder when Anna exploded. Maria handled prevention; Carlos handled crisis management.

They agreed on decision-making rules. For medication decisions (a major conflict area), they agreed that Carlos would raise concerns and Maria would research those concerns thoroughly. They'd discuss findings together and Carlos would make the final call since he'd been more resistant to medication. This gave Carlos input while acknowledging Maria's research skills. For school decisions, Maria made final calls using the same process.

They committed to supporting each other's approaches publicly. When Carlos implemented a new strategy for managing Anna's morning routine, Maria supported it even though she thought it wouldn't work. When Maria's approach later proved more effective, Carlos supported implementing her method without defensiveness.

These changes didn't eliminate all conflict, but they reduced it significantly. More importantly, they helped Maria and Carlos feel like partners again rather than opponents. They reported feeling more connected and less resentful after several months of implementing these strategies.

Communication During Exhaustion

Normal relationship communication advice assumes partners have energy for thoughtful dialogue. Parents of children with DMDD often communicate while exhausted, stressed, and emotionally depleted. This requires different approaches.

Accept that communication will be imperfect and focus on "good enough" rather than ideal. You won't always use "I statements" or avoid defensive reactions. You'll sometimes be short-tempered or impatient. That's reality. Aim for communication that's functional and respectful, not perfect.

Use structured communication formats when discussing difficult topics. One helpful format:

Speaker: States their perspective in two to three sentences max without blaming or criticizing **Listener**: Reflects back what they heard: "I heard you say..." without defending or explaining **Speaker**: Confirms or corrects the reflection **Listener**: Becomes speaker and shares their perspective **Both**: Work toward solution or agree to revisit later

This structure prevents the circular arguments and defensive spirals that happen when both partners are exhausted.

Implement time-outs for heated arguments. Agree in advance that either partner can call a time-out when conversation becomes destructive. The time-out lasts thirty minutes to twenty-four hours (whatever you agree on) and then you return to the discussion. Time-outs prevent saying things you can't take back when stress overrides judgment.

Write notes or emails for complex topics when verbal communication isn't working. Writing allows you to organize thoughts, express yourself without interruption, and give your partner time to process before responding. Emails work well for discussing treatment decisions, expressing concerns, or explaining feelings when face-to-face conversation escalates too quickly.

Use "repair attempts" to reset after conflict. Repair attempts are small gestures that signal you want to reconnect: touching your partner's arm during an argument, making a small joke, saying "I hate fighting with you," or offering an olive branch: "Can we start this conversation over?" Research shows successful couples make and respond to repair attempts during conflict rather than letting arguments spiral.

Practice gratitude even when you're angry. Notice and verbally appreciate things your partner does: "Thank you for getting up with him last night." "I appreciate you handling that insurance call." Gratitude doesn't erase conflict but it prevents relationships from becoming entirely negative.

Separate problem-solving from venting. Sometimes your partner needs solutions; sometimes they need empathy. Ask: "Do you want me to help solve this or just listen?" Trying to solve problems when your partner needs empathy creates frustration. Venting when your partner needs action plan creates different frustration. Clarifying expectations up front helps.

Use abbreviated check-ins when you're too tired for long conversations. A two-minute check-in is better than none: "How are you doing? What's one thing I can do to help you today?" These brief connections maintain minimum relationship maintenance when more isn't possible.

Case Example: The Thompson Family Communication Overhaul

Jason and Michelle Thompson had developed a pattern of attacking each other during disagreements. Both were chronically exhausted from managing their son's DMDD. Their conversations quickly escalated into blame, criticism, and sometimes yelling.

Their couples therapist taught them several communication tools:

They implemented the speaker-listener format for all difficult discussions. At first this felt artificial and slow. But it prevented their usual pattern of interrupting, defending, and escalating. They could actually hear each other's perspectives.

They agreed on a time-out signal—either person could make a "T" shape with their hands and that ended the conversation immediately for one hour. During the time-out, they each did something calming. After the hour, they could continue the conversation or agree it wasn't worth continuing.

They started texting appreciations to each other daily. Jason might text: "Thanks for handling the school meeting. That was hard." Michelle might text: "Appreciate you taking him to therapy so I could rest." These small acknowledgments countered their pattern of only communicating about problems.

They instituted "no DMDD talk" during dinner. Even if dinner lasted only fifteen minutes, they discussed other topics—a show they'd watched, news, memories from before kids. This forced them to connect about something besides their son's condition.

They practiced asking "solve or support?" before launching into advice or empathy. Jason learned that Michelle usually needed him to listen and validate rather than immediately problem-solve. Michelle learned that Jason processed stress by planning solutions and needed her to engage with his ideas rather than just empathizing with his stress.

These tools didn't transform their communication overnight, but they provided structure when exhaustion would have otherwise led to destructive patterns. Both reported feeling more heard and less attacked, which gradually improved their overall relationship quality.

Finding Your Team Again

Beyond managing DMDD effectively, couples need to actively rebuild their identity as partners, not just as co-parents of a child with a challenging disorder.

Prioritize couple time even when it feels impossible. Start small—fifteen minutes of undivided attention matters. Sit together after children sleep and talk about something besides DMDD. Take a walk around the block together. Watch a show you both enjoy. Small moments of connection accumulate into meaningful relationship maintenance.

Work toward occasional longer couple time. Even two hours every other week makes a difference. Use respite care, family help, or trusted babysitters to create space for actual dates. During this time, minimize phone checking and DMDD discussion.

Revive shared interests that existed before DMDD consumed your lives. Did you used to cook together? Try one new recipe monthly. Did you enjoy hiking? Take short hikes when possible. Did you play board games? Pull out those games. Reconnecting with pre-DMDD activities helps you remember who you are as a couple beyond parents-in-crisis.

Create new rituals specific to your current reality. Maybe you can't have elaborate date nights, but you can have coffee together every morning before kids wake. Maybe you can't take vacations, but you can have living room picnics after kids sleep. Rituals that fit your current capacity maintain connection without overwhelming your already taxed resources.

Share laughter intentionally. Humor helps people survive terrible situations. Watch comedy together. Share funny articles. Make jokes. Laughter releases stress, creates positive shared experiences, and reminds you that joy still exists even amidst difficulty.

Express appreciation regularly and specifically. Don't just say "thanks." Say "I appreciate you staying calm when I lost my temper with him today. Your steadiness helps me." Specific appreciation makes your partner feel seen and valued.

Maintain physical affection even if sexual intimacy isn't currently possible. Hold hands. Hug. Sit close on the couch. Physical touch maintains connection and releases oxytocin, which reduces stress and increases bonding. Non-sexual touch is particularly important when sexual intimacy has declined.

Dream together about the future, even if those dreams feel distant. What will you do when your child is more stable? What trips do you want to take eventually? What hobbies do you want to pursue? Dreaming together reminds you that your relationship has a future beyond current crisis and that you're partners in that future.

Seek couples therapy proactively, not as last resort. Couples therapy helps you process the trauma of living with DMDD, develop better communication patterns, resolve resentments before they become relationship-ending, and rebuild connection. Therapy isn't admitting failure—it's accessing support to prevent failure.

Case Example: The Park Family Reclaims Their Relationship

Jennifer and Mike Park spent three years consumed by their daughter's DMDD. By year three, they functioned as efficient crisis managers but no longer felt like a couple. They rarely touched, never laughed, and couldn't recall their last meaningful conversation.

Jennifer suggested couples therapy, which Mike initially resisted. He thought therapy was for relationships that were failing, and he didn't consider their relationship failed—just stressed. Jennifer explained that therapy could help them reconnect before stress caused actual failure. Mike agreed.

The therapist helped them identify what they'd lost: fun, laughter, physical affection, time alone, shared interests. She asked them to each list three small changes they could implement immediately. Jennifer wanted fifteen minutes of couple time nightly and one two-hour date monthly. Mike wanted to restart their tradition of Sunday morning coffee before kids woke and have sex at least twice monthly.

They negotiated. They'd sit together fifteen minutes nightly after their daughter slept, with phones away, just talking. They'd have coffee together every Sunday. They'd try for one four-hour date monthly (more realistic than twice monthly given babysitting challenges). They'd prioritize physical intimacy twice monthly minimum.

They also worked on resentments. Mike resented Jennifer's constant criticism of his parenting. Jennifer resented Mike's habit of checking out emotionally. The therapist helped them express these resentments, understand their sources (Mike felt inadequate; Jennifer felt alone), and develop new patterns.

Six months into therapy, their relationship had improved significantly. They reported feeling like partners again. They laughed together. They looked forward to their Sunday coffee ritual and protected it fiercely. Their sexual intimacy had increased to twice monthly and occasionally more. Most importantly, they felt like a team facing DMDD together rather than two isolated individuals barely surviving.

DMDD challenges marriages in ways few other conditions do. The chronic stress, exhaustion, disagreements, and loss of couple identity create perfect conditions for relationship deterioration. But with intentional effort, clear communication, unified parenting approaches, and commitment to maintaining connection, couples can not only survive DMDD but emerge stronger. Protecting your marriage isn't selfish—it's essential for the entire family's wellbeing. The next chapter addresses another critical but often neglected topic: caregiver self-care and preventing the burnout that threatens your capacity to parent effectively.

Protecting the Partnership Through Crisis

- DMDD creates multiple marriage stressors including chronic stress, exhaustion, different coping styles, treatment disagreements, blame and resentment, loss of shared identity, lack of alone time, absent intimacy, and different grief timelines

- Unified parenting requires agreeing on core principles, developing clear decision-making processes, dividing responsibilities by strengths, creating regular communication routines, presenting united fronts, and supporting each other's approaches

- Exhausted communication needs structured formats, time-outs for heated arguments, written communication for complex topics, repair attempts during conflict, expressed gratitude, separated venting from problem-solving, and brief check-ins when long conversations aren't possible

- Rebuilding couple identity requires prioritizing couple time, reviving shared interests, creating new rituals fitting current capacity, sharing laughter intentionally, expressing specific appreciation, maintaining physical affection, dreaming about future together, and seeking couples therapy proactively

- Protecting marriage isn't selfish but necessary—children need parents who function as partners, not just exhausted individuals managing crisis independently

Chapter 9: Caregiver Self-Care

You're lying awake at 3 AM scrolling through your phone because anxiety won't let you sleep. You've gained thirty pounds from stress eating. You can't remember the last time you did something purely for enjoyment. You declined another invitation from friends because explaining why you can't commit to plans feels too exhausting. You fantasize about running away—not forever, just long enough to sleep without listening for explosions. You're burnt out, depleted, and running on fumes, but you keep going because what choice do you have? Your child needs you. This is the reality of caregiver burnout, and it's destroying you from the inside out.

Recognizing Caregiver Burnout

Burnout differs from regular tiredness or stress. Burnout involves emotional, mental, and physical exhaustion that doesn't improve with rest. It includes cynicism or detachment from work (in this case, parenting), and reduced sense of personal accomplishment or effectiveness. Caregivers of children with DMDD are at extremely high risk for burnout due to the chronic, unpredictable, and intense nature of DMDD symptoms.

Physical signs of burnout include:

- Chronic fatigue that persists despite adequate sleep

- Frequent illness due to weakened immune system

- Changes in appetite (eating much more or much less than usual)

- Sleep problems (insomnia, restless sleep, or sleeping too much)

- Tension headaches or migraines

- Muscle tension, particularly in neck, shoulders, and back

- Digestive problems including stomachaches, nausea, or changes in bowel habits

- Increased substance use (alcohol, prescription medications, caffeine) to cope

Emotional signs of burnout include:

- Feeling emotionally numb or detached

- Loss of motivation or interest in activities previously enjoyed

- Increased irritability or anger

- Feeling helpless, trapped, or defeated

- Detachment or feeling alone in the world

- Decreased satisfaction or sense of accomplishment

- Growing cynical or negative outlook

- Feeling guilty about your negative feelings toward your child

Cognitive signs of burnout include:

- Difficulty concentrating or making decisions

- Memory problems

- Racing thoughts or inability to quiet your mind

- Catastrophic thinking about the future

- Difficulty finding anything positive in situations

- Reduced creativity or problem-solving ability

Behavioral signs of burnout include:

- Withdrawing from friends and family
- Isolating yourself from support systems
- Procrastinating or avoiding responsibilities
- Using food, substances, or other behaviors to cope
- Taking frustrations out on others
- Missing work or calling in sick frequently
- Neglecting personal hygiene or appearance
- Stopping hobbies or activities you used to enjoy

Burnout develops gradually, often so slowly that caregivers don't recognize it until they're in serious crisis. You adapt to worsening symptoms, thinking "this is just how life is now" without realizing you're moving toward complete depletion.

Case Example: Sarah's Breaking Point

Sarah had been managing her son's DMDD for four years. She prided herself on being strong, capable, and dedicated. She attended all appointments, implemented all strategies, and maintained employment despite the chaos. She told everyone she was fine.

She wasn't fine. She'd stopped seeing friends two years ago because she never had energy for social interaction. She gained forty pounds from eating for emotional comfort. She slept poorly, waking multiple times nightly even when her son didn't. She developed chronic tension headaches that required daily pain medication. She cried easily, often breaking down in her car between work and home.

The breaking point came during a routine therapy appointment for her son. The therapist asked how Sarah was doing. Sarah opened her mouth to say "fine" and instead burst into tears. She cried for ten minutes, unable to stop. When she finally calmed enough to speak, she said, "I can't do this anymore. I feel like I'm dying inside."

The therapist recognized severe burnout and insisted Sarah see her own doctor. Sarah's doctor diagnosed her with depression and anxiety, both directly related to chronic caregiver stress. The doctor was blunt: "You cannot continue this way. You're headed toward complete breakdown. Your son needs you, which means you need to take care of yourself immediately."

Sarah resisted. She insisted she didn't have time or energy for self-care. The doctor challenged her: "You'll find time for hospitalization if you collapse completely. Prevention is always less time-consuming than crisis management." This reframing helped Sarah understand that self-care wasn't selfish—it was protective.

Building Your Support Network

Isolation worsens burnout. Connection protects against it. Building and maintaining a support network is necessary, not optional, for caregiver survival.

Identify potential support sources in different categories:

Emotional support comes from people who listen without judgment, validate feelings, and provide empathy. This might include friends, relatives, therapists, support group members, or online community members who understand DMDD.

Practical support comes from people who provide tangible help like childcare, meals, transportation, or assistance with household tasks. This might include family members, neighbors, church members, or paid help.

Informational support comes from people who provide knowledge, advice, or guidance about DMDD, treatment options, school advocacy, or parenting strategies. This includes healthcare providers, therapists, educators, support group facilitators, or experienced DMDD parents.

Companionship support comes from people you spend time with doing non-DMDD-related activities. This includes friends you exercise with, book club members, hobby groups, or anyone who provides social connection beyond your role as DMDD parent.

Most people need support from multiple categories and multiple people. No single person can meet all your support needs. Distribute needs across your support network rather than relying on one or two people who might become overwhelmed.

Actively build support rather than waiting for people to offer:

Be specific about needs when asking for help. Don't say "I could use some help." Say "Could you watch my son for two hours Saturday afternoon so I can go to a yoga class?" Specific requests make it easier for people to say yes and provide the help you actually need.

Accept help when offered even if accepting feels uncomfortable. Many caregivers refuse help out of pride, guilt, or belief they should handle everything independently. This isolation accelerates burnout. Practice saying "yes, that would be helpful" when people offer assistance.

Join support groups specifically for parents of children with behavioral disorders or DMDD. These groups provide connection with people who truly understand your experience. Support groups exist in-person through hospitals or mental health centers and online through social media platforms. The DMDD.org and Revolutionize DMDD websites offer online community connections.

Develop reciprocal relationships where you both give and receive support. Reciprocity makes relationships sustainable. If you only take without giving, people eventually withdraw. If you only give without taking, you deplete yourself further. Balance giving and receiving over time.

Maintain relationships through regular contact even when you don't need immediate help. Check in with friends. Call family members. Attend support group meetings even during calmer periods. Relationships maintained during good times are available during crises.

Use professional support without guilt. Therapists provide support that friends and family can't. They offer expertise, objectivity, and dedicated time focused on your needs. Individual therapy for caregivers provides space to process feelings, develop coping strategies, and prevent burnout.

Case Example: Building Michelle's Support Team

Michelle felt completely alone managing her daughter's DMDD. Her husband worked long hours. Her parents lived across the country. Her friends had drifted away because she'd cancelled plans repeatedly. She felt isolated and unsupported.

Her therapist helped Michelle identify potential support sources and develop a plan to build connections:

Emotional support: Michelle joined an online support group for DMDD parents through Facebook. She connected with three other mothers facing similar challenges. They messaged daily, providing validation and understanding. Michelle also continued individual therapy biweekly.

Practical support: Michelle asked her neighbor if she could watch her daughter occasionally for short periods. The neighbor agreed to two hours monthly. Michelle hired a respite care provider to come four hours twice monthly, giving Michelle time to run errands or rest. She asked her sister to visit one weekend monthly via video call, providing virtual companionship.

Informational support: Michelle attended a parent training program through her daughter's hospital. She connected with the program facilitator who became a resource for questions about strategies and treatment options. She joined a local CHADD chapter where she learned about school advocacy and ADHD management (her daughter had both DMDD and ADHD).

Companionship support: Michelle reconnected with a friend she'd lost touch with, being honest about her situation. The friend suggested they walk together Saturday mornings while Michelle's husband was home with her daughter. Michelle also joined an online book club, giving her something to focus on besides DMDD.

Building this support network took three months of intentional effort. Michelle had to overcome discomfort about asking for help and guilt about taking time for herself. But once the network was established, Michelle felt significantly less isolated. She had people she could text when she needed to vent, people who provided practical breaks, and people who reminded her she had an identity beyond DMDD parent.

Setting Boundaries That Stick

Boundaries protect your limited energy and prevent additional depletion. Many caregivers struggle with boundaries, believing that setting limits is selfish or that they should be available 24/7. This boundary-less approach leads to faster burnout.

Identify necessary boundaries by recognizing what depletes you unnecessarily:

- Do you need boundaries with extended family who offer unwanted advice or criticism?

- Do you need boundaries with schools that call constantly expecting immediate responses?

- Do you need boundaries with friends who don't respect your time or emotional limits?

- Do you need boundaries with your child around certain behaviors or times?

- Do you need boundaries with yourself about perfectionism or self-criticism?

Set boundaries clearly and directly:

- "I need to stop talking about this topic now. Let's discuss something else."

- "I can't take calls before 9 AM. Please text instead if you need something earlier."

- "I'm not available for last-minute requests. Please give me at least 24 hours notice."

- "I need you to stop giving me advice about my child's treatment. I have professionals helping with that."

- "I can help with X, but I can't help with Y."

Enforce boundaries consistently. Setting boundaries means nothing if you don't maintain them. The first time someone pushes against a boundary, restate it clearly. If they continue pushing, implement consequences (ending the conversation, leaving the situation, blocking calls temporarily).

Expect pushback. People accustomed to your boundary-less availability will resist changes. They might call you selfish, unreasonable, or mean. This pushback doesn't mean your boundaries are wrong—it means people don't like adjustments that reduce their access to you. Hold firm anyway.

Practice saying no without over-explaining. "No, that doesn't work for me" is a complete sentence. You don't need to justify or explain every boundary. Over-explaining invites negotiation and makes you feel like you need permission to set limits on your own time and energy.

Implement self-boundaries that protect you from yourself:

- Set a limit on how much time you spend researching DMDD daily

- Establish a bedtime and stick to it even if your mind is racing

- Decide you will not check your child's school portal after 8 PM

- Commit to not criticizing yourself for normal human limitations

- Give yourself permission to feel what you feel without judgment

Create technology boundaries that protect your mental space:

- Turn off school notifications during certain hours

- Remove social media apps if they increase stress

- Set specific times for checking email rather than monitoring constantly

- Put phones away during meals or couple time

- Use "do not disturb" mode liberally

Establish help-seeking boundaries that allow you to accept support:

- Decide it's okay to ask for help even when you could technically handle it alone

- Give yourself permission to hire help rather than doing everything yourself

- Allow others to help even if they don't do things exactly your way

- Accept that needing support doesn't mean you're failing

Case Example: Lisa's Boundary Revolution

Lisa had no boundaries. She answered every call from school immediately, even during work meetings. She accommodated every request from extended family even when those requests were burdensome. She stayed up until 2 AM researching DMDD treatments. She criticized herself constantly for any perceived parenting failure. She was exhausted and resentful.

Her therapist helped Lisa identify necessary boundaries:

School boundary: Lisa told the school she'd respond to non-emergency calls within 24 hours but not immediately. True emergencies could go through her husband's phone. This reduced the constant interruption stress.

Extended family boundary: Lisa's mother-in-law frequently criticized Lisa's parenting choices and offered unsolicited advice. Lisa told her directly: "I appreciate your concern, but I need you to trust that I'm working with professionals who are helping us manage this condition. I need you to stop suggesting alternative approaches." When her mother-in-law persisted, Lisa ended phone calls early and limited visits temporarily.

Research boundary: Lisa limited DMDD research to thirty minutes daily, maximum. After thirty minutes, she closed the computer and did something else. This prevented the spiral of anxiety-driven research that was consuming hours nightly.

Self-criticism boundary: When Lisa noticed self-critical thoughts ("You're a terrible mother," "You should have

130

prevented that explosion"), she practiced responding: "That's not helpful right now. I'm doing my best in an incredibly difficult situation." This internal boundary reduced the constant self-blame.

Help-seeking boundary: Lisa gave herself permission to order takeout twice weekly instead of cooking. She hired a teenager to play with her son for two hours weekly while Lisa did whatever she wanted. She stopped feeling guilty about asking her husband to handle bedtime sometimes even though she "should" be able to do it.

Setting these boundaries initially felt uncomfortable. Lisa worried people would think she was selfish or difficult. Some did push back, particularly her mother-in-law. But over several months, Lisa noticed significant improvements in her stress level, sleep quality, and overall mood. The boundaries protected her energy and created space for minimal self-care.

Finding Moments of Joy

Burnout makes joy feel impossible. Everything is gray, heavy, and difficult. But small moments of joy are both possible and necessary for preventing complete depletion. Joy doesn't have to mean happiness—it can mean brief moments of lightness, pleasure, or peace amidst difficulty.

Identify what brings you joy by asking yourself:

- What did I enjoy before DMDD dominated my life?

- What activities help me feel more like myself?

- What makes me laugh?

- What gives me energy rather than depleting it?

- What helps me feel peaceful or calm?

- What interests me besides my child's condition?

Your answers might include simple things: reading, walking, listening to music, gardening, baking, watching certain shows, talking to specific people, being in nature, exercising, creating art, playing with pets. Joy sources during burnout are often simpler than joy sources during normal life because you have less energy available.

Schedule joy intentionally. Joy doesn't happen accidentally when you're burnt out and overwhelmed. Put it on the calendar. Treat it as seriously as medical appointments. Fifteen minutes of joy daily matters more than waiting for an entire joy-filled day that never comes.

Protect joy time fiercely. Don't let other demands consistently override it. Obviously, genuine emergencies take precedence, but don't let non-emergencies steal time you've designated for joy. Your child's homework battle can wait thirty minutes while you take a walk. The laundry can sit while you read a chapter.

Start small and realistic. Don't aim for hour-long meditation sessions if you haven't meditated in years. Start with two minutes. Don't plan elaborate hobbies requiring significant time investment. Choose activities that fit your current capacity. Brief moments of joy sustained regularly matter more than occasional large doses.

Notice small pleasures throughout your day rather than waiting for big joy experiences:

- The first sip of morning coffee
- Warm sunshine on your face
- Your pet's greeting when you come home
- A song you love coming on the radio
- A text from a friend

- Five minutes of quiet before kids wake

- The feeling after exercise

- A funny meme that makes you laugh

Training yourself to notice these micro-joys helps counter the brain's tendency to focus exclusively on stress and difficulty during burnout. Your brain needs reminders that positive experiences still exist.

Give yourself permission to experience joy without guilt. Many caregivers feel guilty about any moment of enjoyment while their child suffers. But your joy doesn't diminish your child's suffering, and your suffering doesn't reduce your child's suffering. You can be deeply committed to helping your child while also allowing yourself moments of pleasure.

Share joy with others when possible. Joy shared is joy amplified. Watch a comedy with your spouse. Call a friend who makes you laugh. Play with your other children. Dance with your kids to loud music. Shared positive experiences strengthen relationships while providing joy.

Celebrate small victories rather than waiting for major breakthroughs:

- Your child used a coping skill instead of exploding

- You stayed calm during a crisis

- Your family had a good day

- A treatment adjustment is showing promise

- You maintained a boundary successfully

- You did something for yourself without guilt

Acknowledging these small wins trains your brain to notice positive developments rather than fixating exclusively on ongoing challenges.

Case Example: Tom Rebuilds Joy

Tom couldn't remember the last time he felt genuine joy. Managing his daughter's DMDD had consumed everything. He stopped playing guitar, quit his softball league, and dropped his book club membership. He went through motions but felt nothing positive.

His therapist assigned homework: do one thing daily that brought him even a tiny bit of pleasure. Tom protested he didn't have time. The therapist pushed back: "You don't have time not to. Without some positive experiences, you'll burn out completely and be unable to parent at all."

Tom started incredibly small. He listened to one favorite song each morning during his commute. That was all—three minutes of music he enjoyed. After a week, he added five minutes of guitar playing before bed three nights weekly. Another week, he took a ten-minute walk during lunch at work.

These tiny additions didn't transform Tom's life, but they created small pockets of pleasure in otherwise difficult days. After a month, Tom noticed he felt slightly less depleted. He had things to look forward to during hard days—his morning song, evening guitar, lunchtime walk.

Tom gradually expanded his joy activities. He rejoined book club, attending when possible and reading even when he couldn't attend meetings. He started playing softball again, giving himself permission to miss games when family crisis required. He planned a monthly lunch with a friend who made him laugh.

Six months into this process, Tom reported to his therapist: "I still have a daughter with DMDD. Our life is still incredibly hard. But I don't feel like I'm completely drowning anymore. I feel like a person again, not just a crisis manager. Having things I enjoy makes it possible to handle the things that are terrible."

Caregiver self-care isn't selfish indulgence—it's necessary maintenance that protects your capacity to parent through one of the most challenging conditions children face. You cannot pour from an empty cup. You cannot stay regulated if you're completely depleted. You cannot model healthy coping if you're falling apart. Taking care of yourself protects your child by protecting the caregiver they need. This isn't optional—it's survival.

Moving Through Crisis With Intention

Living with DMDD means living with chronic crisis punctuated by acute crises. The strategies in this chapter—recognizing burnout, building support, setting boundaries, and finding joy— don't eliminate the crisis but they help you survive it without being destroyed by it. These strategies protect your mental health, preserve your relationships, and maintain your capacity to keep showing up for your child day after difficult day. Your child needs you whole, not martyred. Your family needs you functional, not depleted. You need yourself healthy, not burnt out beyond recovery. Self-care makes all this possible.

What Caregivers Must Do to Survive

- Burnout involves emotional, mental, and physical exhaustion distinct from normal tiredness, with physical signs like chronic fatigue and illness, emotional signs like detachment and increased irritability, cognitive signs like concentration difficulty, and behavioral signs like isolation and withdrawal

- Support networks require intentional building across emotional, practical, informational, and companionship support categories, with specific requests for help, acceptance of offered assistance, support group participation, and reciprocal relationships maintained through regular contact

- Boundaries protect limited energy through clear identification of unnecessary depletions, direct communication of limits, consistent enforcement despite pushback, practice saying no without over-explaining, self-boundaries preventing self-depletion, technology boundaries protecting mental space, and help-seeking boundaries allowing support acceptance

- Joy must be scheduled intentionally, starting with realistic small moments, protected fiercely from non-emergencies, noticed throughout daily life, experienced without guilt, shared with others when possible, and celebrated through acknowledgment of small victories

- Self-care isn't selfish but necessary survival maintenance protecting caregiver capacity to continue parenting through chronic crisis

Chapter 10: The School System

The principal's email arrives at 10:47 AM requesting an "urgent meeting" about your daughter's behavior. You feel your stomach drop. This is the third urgent meeting this month. You know what's coming—more suspensions, more suggestions that maybe your child would be "better served" elsewhere, more thinly veiled hints that the school can't handle her. You're fighting a system that's supposed to help but often feels like another obstacle standing between your child and the education she deserves.

Building Effective School Partnerships

Schools hold enormous power over your child's daily life and future opportunities. Effective partnerships with school personnel make the difference between your child accessing education or being pushed out. Building these partnerships requires strategy, patience, and consistent effort.

Start before problems escalate. Don't wait for crisis to initiate school contact. Schedule a meeting early in the school year, before major incidents occur, to introduce your child's diagnosis and needs. This proactive approach positions you as a collaborative partner rather than a reactive problem-solver.

During initial meetings, bring documentation including a letter from your child's psychiatrist or psychologist explaining DMDD, how it manifests, what triggers to watch for, and recommended supports. Offer to provide resources about

DMDD that teachers can review. Many educators have never heard of the disorder and genuinely want to understand.

Frame the conversation around partnership. Say things like, "I know my child's behavior creates challenges for you. I want to work together to support his success and make your job easier." This approach acknowledges the teacher's reality while emphasizing shared goals rather than conflicting interests.

Educate without lecturing. Teachers have extensive training in education but limited training in rare psychiatric disorders. Share information about DMDD's neurobiological basis, explaining that your child's brain processes frustration differently. Use accessible language: "Her nervous system treats minor frustrations like major threats. She's not choosing to explode—her alarm system is set too sensitively."

Identify your child's specific patterns so teachers know what to watch for. Does your child shut down during independent work or explode during transitions? Does irritability increase in the afternoon or after lunch? Does your child struggle more with group work or individual tasks? Specific information helps teachers recognize early warning signs and intervene preventively.

Ask what the teacher has noticed. Teachers observe your child in contexts you don't see. They might notice that your child performs better during morning classes, struggles with particular subjects, or responds well to specific teaching styles. This information helps you understand your child more completely and shows the teacher you value their observations.

Maintain regular communication through whatever method works for the teacher. Some prefer email, others like brief phone calls, some use communication notebooks. Weekly check-ins allow you to celebrate successes, address small problems before they become big ones, and maintain relationships beyond crisis management.

Express appreciation specifically. Don't just say "thanks for working with my child." Say "Thank you for giving him extra processing time on that assignment. That accommodation really helped him succeed." Specific appreciation shows you notice their efforts and encourages continued implementation of supports.

Respond to problems promptly but calmly. If the school contacts you about an incident, don't immediately defend your child or attack the school. Say, "Tell me what happened. What can we do to prevent this in the future?" Problem-solving stance builds partnership; defensive stance creates adversaries.

Case Example: The Henderson Partnership Approach

When nine-year-old Tyler Henderson started fourth grade, his mother Elena requested a meeting two weeks into the school year. Tyler had DMDD and a history of explosive incidents at school. Elena brought Tyler's psychiatrist's letter, a one-page DMDD fact sheet, and a list of strategies that had worked in third grade.

During the meeting, Elena said to Tyler's new teacher, Ms. Garcia: "I know Tyler's behavior can be challenging. I appreciate your willingness to work with us. His brain processes frustration differently than other kids, and he hasn't fully developed skills to manage intense emotions. We're working on this in therapy, but he needs support at school too."

Ms. Garcia appreciated Elena's direct approach and asked specific questions about Tyler's triggers. Elena explained that Tyler struggled particularly during math, with transitions, and when he felt corrected in front of peers. Ms. Garcia shared her observations—Tyler seemed most regulated during the first hour of school and became more irritable as the day progressed.

Together, they developed strategies. Ms. Garcia agreed to schedule challenging subjects during Tyler's optimal time, provide five-minute warnings before transitions, and give Tyler corrective feedback privately rather than in front of the class. Elena agreed to email Ms. Garcia briefly every Friday with updates on how Tyler's week went at home and any concerns Elena had noticed.

This partnership approach paid off. When Tyler did have an explosive incident in October, Ms. Garcia contacted Elena to problem-solve rather than simply discipline. They adjusted Tyler's accommodations based on what triggered that incident. By year's end, Tyler's explosive incidents had decreased from weekly to monthly, and Ms. Garcia reported that Tyler had grown significantly in his self-regulation skills.

Documentation Strategies

Documentation protects your child and strengthens your advocacy position. Schools respond to paper trails, data, and formal processes more than verbal requests or emotional appeals.

Document everything from the beginning. Keep a three-ring binder or digital folder containing:

- All communication with school (emails, notes from phone calls, letters)
- Incident reports describing behavioral events
- Copies of all evaluations and assessments
- Medical documentation of your child's diagnosis
- Report cards and progress reports
- Attendance records
- Suspension notices

- Meeting notes from IEP or 504 meetings

Track behavioral incidents systematically. When the school reports an incident, request written documentation. If they provide only verbal information, write it down yourself immediately including date, time, what happened, who was involved, how the school responded, and what consequences occurred.

Track your child's academic performance including grades, test scores, completed assignments, and teacher feedback. If your child's DMDD symptoms affect academic functioning, this documentation proves the connection between the disorder and educational impact.

Track accommodations implementation. If your child has an IEP or 504 Plan, document which accommodations are being implemented and which aren't. Take notes during observations if you visit school. Ask your child regularly which accommodations they're receiving. If accommodations aren't happening, document the gap.

Request copies of all school records annually. Schools must provide your child's educational records within 45 days of your written request. Review these records carefully for accuracy. If you find errors or misleading information, you can request amendments.

Document your requests in writing. Verbal requests carry no legal weight. Put important requests in email or letter form. Request evaluations in writing. Request IEP meetings in writing. Request specific accommodations in writing. Written requests trigger legal timelines that schools must follow.

Keep meeting notes. During IEP or 504 meetings, take detailed notes. Write down who attended, what was discussed, what was decided, and any concerns you raised that weren't addressed.

Send follow-up emails after meetings summarizing agreements and noting any disagreements.

Document your child's strengths alongside problems. Schools often focus exclusively on deficits. Document instances where your child succeeded, used coping skills effectively, showed academic growth, or made social progress. This balanced documentation prevents your child from being defined solely by their struggles.

Create timelines for major issues. If your child has experienced multiple suspensions, create a timeline showing dates, triggers, and outcomes. If you're advocating for increased services, create a timeline showing your requests and the school's responses. Visual timelines help you spot patterns and present information clearly.

Case Example: The Martinez Documentation System

Angela Martinez's son Carlos had DMDD and was facing his fifth suspension in second grade. Angela felt overwhelmed trying to advocate for Carlos while the school insisted his behavior was simply willful defiance. Angela's advocate taught her systematic documentation.

Angela created a three-ring binder with tabbed sections for medical records, school evaluations, behavioral incidents, communication, IEP documents, and Carlos's work samples. She tracked every incident the school reported, requesting written documentation each time. When the school gave only verbal information, Angela sent follow-up emails: "This confirms our phone conversation today where you described that Carlos threw a book during math class at 10:15 AM and received a one-day suspension."

Angela tracked which IEP accommodations Carlos was receiving. She asked Carlos daily which supports his teacher had provided. She discovered that Carlos's IEP specified movement breaks every 30 minutes, but Carlos reported he rarely received these breaks. Angela documented two weeks of Carlos's reports, then emailed the school requesting a meeting to discuss accommodation implementation.

Angela also documented Carlos's successes. She saved work samples showing academic progress. She noted dates Carlos used coping skills successfully. She collected positive notes from his art teacher who reported Carlos thrived in her class.

When Angela finally requested a due process hearing because the school refused to provide adequate support, her documentation proved decisive. She presented a timeline showing twelve months of deteriorating behavior, fourteen documented requests for increased support, and minimal school response. She showed evidence that required accommodations weren't being implemented. She demonstrated that Carlos succeeded when properly supported (shown through art class and home data) but struggled when supports were absent.

The hearing officer ruled in Angela's favor, ordering the school to provide significantly increased services including a one-on-one aide, daily counseling, and comprehensive behavior support. Angela's documentation made her case undeniable.

When Schools Resist Support

Many families encounter school resistance to providing appropriate services. Schools face budget constraints, limited staff, and concerns about setting precedents. Understanding resistance sources helps you develop effective counter-strategies.

Common resistance tactics schools use:

Minimizing the problem: "He's doing fine academically. His grades are passing." Response: "His grades don't reflect his potential, and he's experiencing significant emotional distress daily. The law doesn't require failure before providing support—

it requires support when disability affects educational performance."

Blaming home environment: "This behavior only happens at school. Maybe there are issues at home we should address first." Response: "His psychiatrist has diagnosed a neurological condition that affects emotional regulation. The home environment doesn't cause DMDD. He may show more symptoms at home because school demands exhaust his regulatory capacity, but the disorder is consistent across settings."

Suggesting alternative placements: "Perhaps your child would do better in a smaller setting or alternative school." Response: "Federal law requires you to provide appropriate services in the least restrictive environment. That means here, with proper support, unless you're stating that you cannot provide FAPE (free appropriate public education) in this setting."

Claiming budget limitations: "We'd love to provide that service, but we don't have the resources." Response: "Budget concerns cannot override my child's legal rights. If you lack resources to provide FAPE, that's a district problem to solve, not a reason to deny appropriate services."

Offering minimal services: "We can give him one 30-minute counseling session per month." Response: "Based on his psychiatrist's recommendations and the severity of his needs, monthly counseling is insufficient. I'm requesting the evaluation team determine appropriate service levels based on his needs, not on what's typically available."

Delaying evaluations or meetings: "We're very busy. We can schedule that meeting in six weeks." Response: "Federal law requires you to respond to my written evaluation request within a specific timeframe. I'm requesting written confirmation of when evaluation will begin and when the meeting will occur."

When schools actively resist, escalate through proper channels:

1. Document the resistance including dates of requests, school responses, and specific services denied or delayed.

2. Request clarification in writing. Email: "I'm requesting written explanation of why you're denying the accommodation recommended by my child's psychiatrist."

3. Bring an advocate to meetings. Advocates know the law and can challenge illegal resistance directly.

4. File complaints with your state education department if schools violate procedural requirements (missing timelines, refusing evaluations, denying meetings).

5. Request mediation to resolve disputes with neutral third-party facilitator.

6. Initiate due process if other approaches fail. Due process is formal legal proceeding where hearing officer decides disputes.

7. Contact OCR (Office for Civil Rights) if you believe discrimination is occurring based on disability.

Case Example: The Robinson Family Battles School Resistance

The Robinson family fought for two years to get appropriate services for their daughter Maya, who had DMDD. The school insisted Maya was "just having behavior problems" and needed stricter discipline rather than special education services.

The Robinsons requested evaluation in writing. The school delayed six months before beginning evaluation, then concluded Maya didn't qualify for an IEP because her grades were passing. The Robinsons disagreed and requested an Independent Educational Evaluation (IEE) at school expense. The school refused.

The Robinsons filed a state complaint about the delayed evaluation timeline and the refusal to provide an IEE. The state found in their favor on both issues, ordering the school to conduct a new evaluation immediately and fund an independent evaluation.

The independent evaluator found Maya clearly qualified under "emotional disturbance" category. Her DMDD significantly affected her ability to learn and maintain relationships. The evaluator recommended extensive services including daily counseling, behavior support plan, crisis intervention services, and numerous classroom accommodations.

The school resisted implementing these recommendations, offering only weekly counseling. The Robinsons requested mediation. During mediation, their advocate presented three years of documentation showing Maya's escalating symptoms, fourteen suspension notices, declining academic performance despite average intelligence, and the school's repeated refusals to provide support.

The school finally agreed to implement most recommended services. Within one school year of receiving appropriate support, Maya's suspensions stopped, her grades improved from Cs and Ds to As and Bs, and her parents reported significant improvement in her overall functioning.

Alternative Educational Options

Sometimes, despite all efforts, traditional public school doesn't work for children with DMDD. Alternative options exist, each with advantages and limitations.

Charter schools are public schools operating independently of traditional district control. Some charter schools specialize in students with behavioral or emotional challenges. Advantages include smaller class sizes, specialized approaches, and flexibility. Limitations include enrollment lotteries, transportation challenges if outside your district, and variable quality.

Private schools offer more individualized attention but require tuition (often $15,000-$40,000 annually). Some private schools specialize in students with learning or emotional challenges. Few private schools have legal obligations to provide services like public schools do. Some states offer scholarship programs helping families afford private school for children with disabilities.

Therapeutic day schools serve students with significant emotional or behavioral disorders, providing both education and intensive therapeutic support. These schools have mental health professionals on staff, small class sizes, and expertise managing challenging behaviors. Students often need IEP placement in therapeutic day school, meaning the public school district pays tuition if they cannot provide FAPE in less restrictive settings.

Online schooling allows students to complete work from home at their own pace. This option removes peer interaction stressors and allows flexible scheduling around therapy appointments and difficult days. Limitations include lack of socialization, need for parent involvement, and limited access to real-time teacher support.

Homeschooling gives families complete control over curriculum, pace, and structure. Parents can build in breaks, adjust to their child's regulatory capacity, and eliminate triggers present in school environments. Challenges include time commitment (a parent must be available), lack of socialization opportunities, missing out on school-provided services, and financial strain if a parent must leave employment to homeschool.

Hybrid models combine approaches. Some students attend school part-time (mornings only when they're most regulated) and complete work at home for remaining subjects. Some families homeschool with supplemental services provided by the school district. Some students use online curriculum for certain subjects while attending traditional school for others.

Residential treatment serves students with severe symptoms requiring 24-hour care. These programs provide intensive therapy, psychiatric care, and education on campus. Residential treatment is appropriate when students pose ongoing safety risks that cannot be managed in home or community settings. Insurance or school districts may fund residential treatment when medically or educationally necessary.

Determining the right placement requires honest assessment:

- Can your child access learning in their current setting with appropriate accommodations?

- Are behavioral symptoms so severe that they prevent learning despite supports?

- Is the current setting causing trauma or significantly worsening symptoms?

- What setting would allow your child to make meaningful progress?

- What resources (financial, time, support) does your family have available?

Case Example: Three Families, Three Different Choices

The Kim Family—Therapeutic Day School: The Kims' daughter Sophia attended public school through fourth grade despite significant struggles. By fifth grade, Sophia was suspended monthly for explosive behavior, academically failing, and becoming increasingly depressed. The school refused to provide adequate support.

The Kims requested that Sophia's IEP team consider therapeutic day school placement. After extensive evaluation, the team agreed Sophia needed more support than the public school could provide. The district placed Sophia in a therapeutic day school 15 miles away.

At the therapeutic day school, Sophia had eight students in her class, two staff members (a teacher and counselor), daily individual therapy, and a behavior support plan implemented consistently. The school had crisis intervention protocols and sensory spaces. After one year, Sophia's explosive incidents decreased dramatically, her academic performance improved, and she reported feeling supported rather than punished for her symptoms.

The Chen Family—Homeschooling: The Chens pulled their son Marcus from school midyear after his third hospitalization for suicidal ideation following ongoing bullying related to his DMDD symptoms. The school environment had become traumatic for Marcus.

Marcus's mother quit her job to homeschool. They used online curriculum allowing Marcus to work at his own pace. They scheduled schoolwork during Marcus's optimal regulation times (mornings) and kept sessions brief (30-45 minutes with breaks). Marcus attended weekly therapy and a homeschool co-op for socialization.

Homeschooling allowed Marcus to heal from school trauma without the pressure of daily peer interaction. After 18 months, Marcus's symptoms improved significantly. The family re-enrolled Marcus in public school for eighth grade with robust supports in place, and he successfully completed middle school and high school.

The Torres Family—Hybrid Model: The Torres family negotiated a hybrid arrangement for their daughter Ana. Ana attended school from 8 AM to 11:30 AM when her regulation was strongest. She participated in English, social studies, and electives. She completed math and science at home using online curriculum.

This arrangement reduced the regulatory demands on Ana while maintaining peer interaction and school connection. The half-day schedule meant Ana had energy left after school for therapy appointments and family time. She avoided the after-lunch deterioration that had triggered most of her previous explosive incidents.

The hybrid model continued through seventh and eighth grade. By ninth grade, Ana's symptoms had improved enough that she attended full days with continued accommodations. The hybrid years allowed Ana to stay connected to school while reducing stress to manageable levels during a difficult developmental period.

Schools hold enormous power over your child's daily experiences and long-term opportunities. Effective school partnerships, strong documentation, strategies for managing resistance, and knowledge of alternative options give you tools to ensure your child receives the education they deserve despite the challenges DMDD presents. The school system is just one part of the network of support your child needs—the healthcare system provides another, with its own set of challenges and strategies for success.

What You Need to Navigate Schools Successfully

- Effective partnerships require proactive communication, education about DMDD, identification of specific patterns, regular contact, expressed appreciation, and problem-solving stance during conflicts

- Documentation protects your child through systematic tracking of incidents, academic performance, accommodation implementation, formal written requests, detailed meeting notes, and balanced recording of both struggles and successes

- School resistance manifests through minimizing problems, blaming home environment, suggesting alternative placements, claiming budget limitations, offering minimal services, or delaying evaluations—counter with knowledge of legal rights and escalation through complaints, mediation, or due process when necessary

- Alternative options include charter schools, private schools, therapeutic day schools, online schooling, homeschooling, hybrid models, or residential treatment—each with different advantages and limitations requiring honest assessment of child needs and family resources

Chapter 11: Healthcare and Insurance

Your insurance company denied coverage for your son's psychiatric hospitalization—$18,000 you don't have. The denial letter uses phrases like "not medically necessary" despite your son's psychiatrist saying the hospitalization was essential. You have three days to file an appeal. Meanwhile, you're trying to find a psychiatrist who specializes in DMDD, accepts your insurance, and has openings before 2027. The healthcare system feels deliberately designed to prevent access to care.

Finding Specialized Care

DMDD requires specialized treatment, but finding providers with DMDD expertise presents significant challenges. The disorder is relatively new (added to DSM-5 in 2013), meaning many clinicians completed training before DMDD existed as a recognized diagnosis.

Start with your child's pediatrician for referrals to child psychiatrists and psychologists in your area. Pediatricians maintain networks of specialists and know which providers accept various insurance plans.

Contact major children's hospitals in your region. Academic medical centers typically have child psychiatry departments with specialists in complex mood disorders. They may have longer wait times but offer expertise hard to find elsewhere.

Call your insurance company for lists of in-network child psychiatrists and psychologists. When calling providers on the list, ask specifically: "Do you have experience treating Disruptive Mood Dysregulation Disorder?" Many providers won't, but some will have treated the symptoms even if they're not familiar with the specific diagnosis.

Use online directories including:

- Psychology Today therapist finder

- American Academy of Child and Adolescent Psychiatry provider database

- CHADD professional directory

- State psychological association referral services

Search for providers treating related conditions. If you can't find DMDD specialists, look for providers specializing in "pediatric mood disorders," "childhood irritability and aggression," or "explosive behavior in children." Providers treating these issues likely have relevant expertise.

Contact DMDD-focused organizations including DMDD.org and Revolutionize DMDD (rdmdd.org). These organizations maintain provider directories and can connect families with clinicians experienced in treating DMDD.

Ask about treatment approaches when interviewing potential providers. Look for familiarity with evidence-based treatments including cognitive behavioral therapy, dialectical behavior therapy adapted for children, parent training, and medication management. Providers should know about the Matthews Protocol or at least be willing to learn about emerging treatments.

Consider telehealth if local options are limited. Many states now allow licensed mental health providers to treat patients via video conference across state lines. Telehealth expands your provider options significantly.

Plan for wait times. Child psychiatrists are in short supply nationally. Average wait times range from 6 weeks to 6 months for initial appointments. Get on multiple waiting lists simultaneously. Call regularly to check for cancellations.

Build a treatment team rather than relying on a single provider. Your child likely needs:

- A child psychiatrist for medication management
- A therapist (psychologist, clinical social worker, or counselor) for weekly therapy
- A parent training program leader for caregiver support
- School-based counselor or psychologist for in-school support
- Primary care pediatrician coordinating medical care

Team-based care ensures comprehensive treatment addressing multiple needs simultaneously.

Case Example: The Williams Family's Three-Year Search

The Williams family lived in a rural area 90 minutes from the nearest children's hospital. When their daughter Emma was diagnosed with DMDD at age seven, their pediatrician gave them a list of three child psychiatrists. All three had 6-month wait lists. The Williams got on all three lists.

After waiting six months, Emma saw a psychiatrist who admitted she'd never treated DMDD specifically but had experience with childhood mood disorders. The psychiatrist prescribed medications that helped moderately but not dramatically. After nine months with minimal progress, the Williams sought a second opinion.

They expanded their search to include providers two hours away. They contacted the children's hospital in the nearest city. The hospital had a specialized mood disorders clinic, and one psychiatrist there had treated several DMDD cases. The wait list was four months.

While waiting, Emma's mother joined an online DMDD parent support group. Another parent mentioned a psychiatrist in a neighboring state who provided telehealth consultations and specialized in treatment-resistant childhood mood disorders. The Williams contacted this psychiatrist.

The telehealth psychiatrist reviewed Emma's records and recommended the Matthews Protocol, which Emma's local psychiatrist wasn't familiar with. The telehealth psychiatrist consulted with Emma's local psychiatrist, explaining the protocol. Emma's local psychiatrist agreed to implement it under the specialist's guidance.

This collaboration proved successful. Emma's symptoms improved significantly on the Matthews Protocol. The Williams maintained quarterly telehealth consultations with the specialist while the local psychiatrist managed day-to-day medication adjustments. By combining local care with remote expertise, they accessed specialized treatment despite geographic barriers.

Navigating Insurance Denials

Insurance companies frequently deny mental health treatment claims, sometimes for legitimate reasons but often using tactics that violate federal mental health parity laws requiring equal coverage for mental and physical health conditions.

Common denial reasons include:

"Not medically necessary": Insurance claims treatment isn't needed despite provider recommendation. This often occurs with hospitalizations, intensive outpatient programs, or frequent therapy.

"Experimental or investigational": Insurance refuses to cover treatments they claim lack sufficient research support. This often affects newer approaches like the Matthews Protocol.

"Out of network": Insurance denies coverage because you used a provider outside their network, even if no in-network providers were available or appropriate.

"Prior authorization not obtained": Insurance denies because you didn't get pre-approval, even if the treatment was emergency or you didn't know pre-authorization was required.

"Maximum benefits exceeded": Insurance claims you've hit your coverage limit, even when such limits are illegal under mental health parity laws.

Understanding your rights:

Mental health parity laws require insurance companies to cover mental health and substance use disorder treatment at the same level they cover medical/surgical care. They can't impose stricter limits on mental health coverage.

Appeals processes give you the right to challenge denials. Insurance companies must explain denial reasons and your appeal rights in denial letters. Most plans allow at least two levels of appeal—internal review by the insurance company and external review by independent third party.

Emergency treatment must be covered even if provided out-of-network or without prior authorization. If your child required psychiatric hospitalization due to safety concerns, insurance cannot deny coverage because you didn't get pre-approval during the crisis.

Steps to fight denials:

1. Request detailed explanation of denial including specific policy language supporting the denial and clinical criteria used to determine treatment wasn't necessary.

2. Gather supporting documentation including letter from your child's provider explaining why treatment is medically necessary, clinical notes documenting symptom severity, research supporting the treatment approach, and documentation of lack of in-network alternatives if relevant.

3. File internal appeal within the timeframe specified in your denial letter (usually 180 days). Submit all supporting documentation and a detailed letter explaining why the denial was wrong.

4. Request expedited appeal if delay in treatment will cause serious harm to your child's health. Expedited appeals must be decided within 72 hours.

5. File external review if internal appeal is denied. External review goes to independent medical reviewer who makes binding decision.

6. Contact your state insurance commissioner to file a complaint if you believe the insurance company violated state law or mental health parity requirements.

7. Consult an attorney specializing in healthcare law if the denial involves large amounts of money or ongoing treatment denials. Some attorneys work on contingency (no fee unless you win).

8. Use your employer's help if you have employer-sponsored insurance. HR departments can pressure insurance companies to reverse improper denials because the employer is the actual customer.

Case Example: The Martinez Insurance Battle

The Martinez family's son Diego required psychiatric hospitalization after becoming acutely suicidal. Diego stayed in the hospital 12 days while his treatment team stabilized medications and ensured his safety. The hospital bill totaled $22,000.

Two months later, the Martinez family received a letter from their insurance company denying coverage for the entire hospitalization. The denial claimed the hospitalization was "not medically necessary" and could have been handled at a "lower level of care."

Diego's mother, Carmen, was furious. The hospital psychiatrist had documented daily that Diego remained actively suicidal and unsafe for discharge. Carmen gathered documentation including:

- Admission note documenting Diego's suicide attempt and plan

- Daily progress notes showing ongoing suicidal ideation

- Safety assessment showing Diego couldn't be safely treated outpatient

- Discharge summary explaining 12 days were necessary to achieve stability

- Letter from Diego's outpatient psychiatrist stating hospitalization was essential

Carmen filed an internal appeal including all documentation and a detailed letter explaining that denying coverage for emergency psychiatric care for an actively suicidal child violated both common sense and mental health parity laws.

The insurance company denied the internal appeal, again claiming hospitalization exceeded what was "medically necessary." Carmen filed an external review with an independent reviewer and simultaneously filed complaints with her state insurance commissioner and the U.S. Department of Labor (her insurance was through her husband's employer).

The external reviewer, a child psychiatrist not affiliated with the insurance company, reviewed all documentation and ruled entirely in the Martinez family's favor. The reviewer stated clearly that the hospitalization was not only medically necessary but was standard appropriate care for a child with Diego's symptoms.

The insurance company was required to pay the full claim. Additionally, the state insurance commissioner investigated and found the company had systematically denied mental health claims at higher rates than medical claims, violating parity laws. The company faced fines and had to review and reprocess numerous other denied mental health claims.

Hospitalization Timeline and Expectations

Psychiatric hospitalization for children is traumatic for families but sometimes necessary when safety cannot be maintained outpatient. Understanding what to expect reduces anxiety and helps you advocate effectively during the process.

When hospitalization becomes necessary:

- Child is actively suicidal with plan and intent
- Child is homicidal or has seriously injured others
- Child's behavior poses imminent danger to self or others that cannot be managed at home or outpatient
- Child requires medication adjustments or diagnostic clarification that cannot be done safely outpatient

- Child has become completely non-functional and family can no longer provide care

How hospitalization happens:

Emergency department route: Most hospitalizations begin in a hospital emergency department. You bring your child (or they're brought by ambulance or police) to the ED. The ED conducts medical clearance ensuring no physical health issues are causing psychiatric symptoms. A psychiatrist or psychiatric social worker evaluates your child to determine if hospitalization is warranted.

ED waits can be long—6 to 24 hours is common. Bring your child's medication list, current prescribers' contact information, and any documentation of the current crisis. Stay calm even if you're terrified. Your child needs you to be their steady presence during a scary experience.

Direct admission route: If your child's outpatient psychiatrist has admitting privileges at a psychiatric hospital, they might arrange direct admission bypassing the ED. This is faster and less traumatic but not always available.

Involuntary commitment: If your child refuses hospitalization and meets criteria for being danger to self or others, they can be hospitalized involuntarily. Each state has different commitment laws and procedures. Involuntary commitment typically requires court hearing within 72 hours determining if continued hospitalization is warranted.

What happens during hospitalization:

Admission process: Staff complete extensive paperwork, conduct searches for safety (removing any items that could be used for self-harm), and orient your child to the unit. Your child will likely be frightened. Unit staff are experienced helping scared children adjust.

Daily schedule: Most units have structured schedules including group therapy, individual therapy, school/educational time, recreation, meals, and medication times. Visitors are typically allowed during specific hours.

Treatment team: Your child's team includes an attending psychiatrist, social worker, nurses, mental health techs, and sometimes occupational therapist, recreation therapist, and education staff. The team meets regularly to discuss your child's progress.

Medication management: The primary focus is often stabilizing medications. The psychiatrist may adjust current medications, try new medications, or discontinue medications that aren't working. Close monitoring in hospital allows faster medication changes than possible outpatient.

Safety: Hospitalization provides 24-hour safety monitoring. Staff check on patients frequently. Bedrooms have minimal furniture and no items that could be used for self-harm. This level of safety isn't possible at home.

Family involvement: Most programs include family therapy sessions and family meetings with the treatment team. Your input is crucial. Be honest about what's happening at home, what's working, and what isn't.

Discharge planning: The team begins discharge planning from day one. They'll work with you to arrange follow-up appointments, adjust home safety plans, implement school accommodations, and ensure you have resources needed for successful transition home.

Average length of stay: Most children stay 5 to 14 days. Length depends on symptom severity, response to treatment, insurance coverage, and availability of appropriate discharge resources.

After discharge, expect:

- Intense follow-up appointments (often within 72 hours of discharge)

- Possible continued medication adjustments

- Your child may feel emotional about the experience

- Siblings may need support processing what happened

- School re-entry may require planning and accommodations

Case Example: The Thompson Hospitalization Experience

Ten-year-old Aiden Thompson's DMDD symptoms escalated to the point where he was threatening to kill himself daily and had tried to run into traffic twice. His parents brought him to the emergency department.

The ED wait lasted eight hours. Aiden was frightened and angry, alternating between crying and raging. His parents stayed calm, explained what was happening in simple terms, and reassured Aiden that the hospital would help him feel safer.

Finally, a psychiatrist evaluated Aiden. The evaluation took 90 minutes. The psychiatrist agreed hospitalization was necessary. Aiden was admitted to the child psychiatric unit around 2 AM.

During his 10-day stay, Aiden initially refused to participate in groups and was hostile toward staff. By day three, he began engaging. The psychiatrist made significant medication changes, implementing the Matthews Protocol that Aiden's outpatient psychiatrist had been reluctant to try.

Aiden's parents visited daily during visiting hours. They attended two family therapy sessions and one family team meeting. The social worker helped them understand Aiden's triggers better and taught them new de-escalation techniques.

By day eight, Aiden was calmer and reported feeling less suicidal. The team began discharge planning. They scheduled an appointment with Aiden's outpatient psychiatrist for two days post-discharge. They adjusted Aiden's IEP accommodations. They created a detailed safety plan for home.

Aiden discharged on day 10. The first week home was rocky— Aiden felt embarrassed about the hospitalization and worried peers would find out. His parents worked with the school to develop a re-entry plan that protected Aiden's privacy.

Three months post-hospitalization, the medication changes made during the hospital stay were still helping significantly. Aiden's suicidal ideation had resolved. While he still had DMDD symptoms, they were more manageable. Aiden's mother told their therapist, "The hospitalization was terrifying, but it probably saved his life. The intensive intervention broke the crisis cycle we couldn't break on our own."

Building Your Medical Team

Effective DMDD treatment requires a coordinated medical team rather than a single provider. Building and maintaining this team requires intentional effort.

Your team should include:

Pediatrician or family doctor: Your child's primary care provider coordinates general medical care, monitors physical health, prescribes treatment for medical illnesses, and serves as the entry point for specialist referrals.

Child psychiatrist: Manages psychiatric medications, monitors for side effects, adjusts medications based on response, provides diagnostic clarification, and coordinates with other mental health providers.

Therapist (psychologist, clinical social worker, licensed professional counselor): Provides weekly individual therapy teaching coping skills, processes difficult experiences, monitors safety, and coordinates with psychiatrist regarding overall treatment.

Parent trainer or family therapist: Teaches caregivers effective strategies for managing behavior, preventing escalation, and responding to crises. Family therapy addresses how DMDD affects family functioning.

School psychologist or counselor: Provides in-school support, implements behavior plans, participates in IEP meetings, and monitors academic and social functioning.

Specialized evaluators: Neuropsychologists assess cognitive functioning and learning differences. Occupational therapists assess sensory processing. Educational evaluators assess academic skills.

Coordination is key:

Sign release forms allowing your providers to communicate with each other. Many clinicians default to not communicating without explicit permission. Releases enable information sharing that improves treatment.

Request provider communication explicitly. Say to your psychiatrist: "Can you please call my child's therapist to coordinate medication changes with what they're seeing in therapy?" Most providers will communicate if asked.

Share information across providers. If your child's teacher reports something important, share it with your psychiatrist and therapist. If your psychiatrist changes medications, inform your pediatrician and therapist.

Schedule periodic team meetings where all providers join one meeting (in-person or by phone) to discuss your child's progress and adjust treatment collaboratively. Most providers will participate in 30-minute team meetings if properly scheduled.

Be the coordinator. As the parent, you're the only person who sees all aspects of your child's life and treatment. You must actively ensure providers communicate rather than assuming they will independently.

Keep everyone informed of significant changes including medication changes, school problems, family stressors, symptom changes, or hospitalization.

Resolve conflicts between providers directly. If your therapist recommends one approach and your psychiatrist recommends something different, facilitate a conversation between them rather than being caught in the middle.

Case Example: The Chen Family's Coordinated Team

The Chen family's daughter Mei had DMDD, ADHD, and anxiety. Her treatment team included a pediatrician, child psychiatrist, psychologist providing weekly therapy, parent trainer running their parent management program, and school psychologist.

Initially, these providers worked in silos. The psychiatrist prescribed medications without knowing what the therapist was observing. The therapist taught coping skills without knowing about medication side effects. The school psychologist implemented behavior plans without input from mental health providers.

Mei's mother, Lin, recognized this lack of coordination was limiting Mei's progress. Lin signed releases allowing all providers to communicate. She requested the psychiatrist and therapist have a phone conversation to coordinate care. She shared the therapist's progress notes with the psychiatrist and vice versa.

Lin scheduled a team meeting including all providers. During the 45-minute video conference, the team reviewed Mei's current functioning, discussed what was working and what wasn't, and developed a coordinated treatment plan.

The psychiatrist learned from the therapist that Mei's current medication was causing afternoon irritability that worsened DMDD symptoms. The psychiatrist adjusted the medication schedule. The therapist learned from the psychiatrist about side effects to watch for. The school psychologist learned from both about strategies to implement at school. The parent trainer incorporated insights from all providers into recommendations for home management.

After implementing the coordinated plan, Mei's progress accelerated. Problems got addressed quickly because providers communicated regularly. Strategies were consistent across settings. Everyone worked toward shared goals instead of potentially contradictory approaches.

Lin continued coordinating team meetings quarterly and facilitated phone calls between providers whenever significant changes occurred. She considered this coordination part of her parental responsibility—ensuring all the experts helping her daughter actually worked together as a team.

The healthcare system creates barriers to accessing appropriate treatment for DMDD through provider shortages, insurance denials, and fragmented care. But with knowledge of how to find specialized care, strategies for fighting insurance denials, understanding of hospitalization processes, and commitment to building coordinated treatment teams, families can navigate these barriers successfully. The medical support your child receives now shapes their trajectory as they grow older and face new developmental challenges, which brings us to the adolescent years and beyond.

Navigating Healthcare Successfully

- Finding specialized care requires creative searching including pediatrician referrals, children's hospitals, insurance directories, online resources, DMDD-focused organizations, telehealth options, and building complete treatment teams rather than relying on single providers

- Insurance denials can be fought through understanding mental health parity laws, requesting detailed denial explanations, gathering provider documentation, filing internal appeals, requesting expedited reviews when necessary, filing external reviews, and contacting state regulators or attorneys when companies violate laws

- Hospitalization provides safety and intensive intervention when outpatient care becomes insufficient, with typical stays of 5-14 days including medication stabilization, therapy, discharge planning, and intensive follow-up care post-discharge

- Medical teams work best when coordinated through signed release forms, explicit requests for provider communication, information sharing across team members, periodic team meetings, parent coordination of all providers, and direct conflict resolution between providers

Chapter 12: Adolescence and Beyond

Your son turned thirteen last week. You've been managing his DMDD since he was seven. You thought you understood this disorder inside and out. Then the explosions that used to last thirty minutes now last two hours. The irritability that was manageable with strategies now includes substance use. The sadness you occasionally noticed has become pervasive depression with suicidal thoughts. Adolescence has changed everything, and you're back at the beginning trying to figure out this new version of the disorder you thought you knew.

How DMDD Changes With Age

DMDD is diagnosed between ages 6 and 18, but the disorder doesn't look the same across this entire age range. Research shows that as children with DMDD reach adolescence and young adulthood, the disorder often shifts in presentation and sometimes diagnosis.

Early adolescence (ages 11-14) often sees:

- Physical size increasing, making explosive behavior more dangerous

- Verbal aggression becoming more sophisticated and cutting

- Property destruction involving more valuable items (phones, computers, furniture)

- Peer conflicts increasing as social dynamics become more complex

- Academic demands intensifying, creating more frustration triggers

- Hormonal changes affecting mood regulation

- Greater awareness of being "different" from peers, leading to shame and isolation

Mid-adolescence (ages 15-17) typically shows:

- Explosive temper outbursts decreasing in frequency but not necessarily intensity

- Chronic irritability persisting or worsening

- Depression symptoms emerging or intensifying

- Anxiety disorders developing

- Substance use beginning as self-medication

- Suicidal ideation or behaviors increasing

- Family conflict intensifying around independence issues

- School disengagement or refusal

Late adolescence and young adulthood (ages 18-25) research indicates:

- DMDD diagnosis no longer applies (age limit is 18)

- Many individuals develop major depressive disorder

- Anxiety disorders common

- Some develop bipolar disorder, though this is less common than previously thought

- Functional impairment continuing including difficulties with employment, relationships, and independent living

- Higher rates of substance use disorders

- Increased risk for physical health problems

- Lower educational attainment compared to peers

The transformation isn't universal. Some adolescents with childhood DMDD see significant symptom reduction as their brains mature and they develop better coping skills. Others experience worsening symptoms. Still others shift from external explosions to internal symptoms like depression and anxiety. Predicting individual trajectories remains difficult.

What drives these changes:

Brain development: The adolescent brain undergoes massive restructuring, particularly in the prefrontal cortex (responsible for impulse control and emotional regulation) and limbic system (involved in emotional processing). This normal developmental process can temporarily worsen emotional dysregulation before eventual improvement.

Hormonal changes: Puberty brings dramatic hormonal shifts affecting mood, sleep, stress responses, and emotional reactivity. These changes can exacerbate DMDD symptoms.

Social demands: Adolescent social worlds become more complex, judgmental, and high-stakes. Children with DMDD often struggle with peer relationships, leading to increased isolation, bullying, and social rejection that worsen mood symptoms.

Academic pressures: High school academic demands increase significantly. Adolescents with DMDD who have difficulty with frustration tolerance struggle with complex assignments, time management, and increased homework loads.

Identity development: Adolescents naturally question who they are and develop independent identities. Adolescents with DMDD often incorporate their disorder into their identity, seeing themselves as "broken" or "bad," which contributes to depression and hopelessness.

Treatment responsiveness: Adolescents can benefit from more sophisticated therapy approaches than younger children. Cognitive behavioral therapy, dialectical behavior therapy, and insight-oriented therapy become more effective as teens develop abstract thinking capabilities. However, adolescent resistance to treatment also increases—teens may refuse medication, skip therapy, or engage in treatment-interfering behaviors.

Case Example: Marcus's Adolescent Transformation

Marcus was diagnosed with DMDD at age eight. Throughout elementary school, he had frequent explosive tantrums— screaming, throwing objects, hitting walls—but these episodes were short-lived and he'd calm with parental support.

When Marcus hit puberty at age twelve, everything changed. His tantrums became less frequent but longer and more intense. A tantrum that used to last twenty minutes now lasted two hours. Marcus destroyed his bedroom twice, putting fist-sized holes in walls and breaking furniture. His parents felt genuinely afraid during his rages because Marcus was now their size and stronger than his mother.

Marcus's chronic irritability worsened significantly. He went from being grumpy most days to being hostile and angry nearly all the time. He snapped at everyone, isolated himself in his room, and refused to participate in family activities. His grades dropped from Bs and Cs to Ds and Fs. Teachers reported Marcus was disengaged and uncooperative.

By age fourteen, Marcus's explosive outbursts had decreased— not because his emotional regulation improved but because his symptoms shifted inward. He stopped exploding at others and started destroying himself. He developed significant depression, spending days in bed refusing to go to school. He began cutting himself. He told his therapist he thought about suicide daily.

Marcus's psychiatrist adjusted his diagnosis to include major depressive disorder alongside DMDD. Treatment shifted to focus more on depression while continuing to address emotional dysregulation. Marcus started an antidepressant medication and intensive outpatient therapy program.

The adolescent years were brutal for Marcus and his family. But by age sixteen, with consistent treatment, Marcus began stabilizing. He still struggled with depression and irritability, but he developed better insight into his symptoms and more willingness to use coping strategies. His parents described it as "emerging from a nightmare into something manageable."

The Anxiety and Depression Connection

Research consistently shows that children with DMDD face dramatically increased risk for developing anxiety disorders and major depression as they reach adolescence and young adulthood. Understanding this connection helps families recognize emerging symptoms early and seek appropriate treatment.

Depression develops frequently in adolescents who had childhood DMDD. One major longitudinal study found that young adults with childhood DMDD history had seven times the rate of depression compared to peers without DMDD history. Another study found that 50 percent of adolescents with DMDD developed major depressive disorder within 3 years.

Why the depression connection:

Chronic stress: Living with DMDD means years of emotional distress, social struggles, family conflict, and academic challenges. This chronic stress affects brain development and increases depression vulnerability.

Learned helplessness: After years of trying to control their emotions and repeatedly failing, children with DMDD often develop learned helplessness—belief that they cannot control what happens to them. This thinking pattern strongly predicts depression.

Social isolation: DMDD symptoms damage peer relationships. By adolescence, many children with DMDD have few or no friends. Social isolation is one of the strongest depression risk factors.

Negative self-concept: Children with DMDD receive enormous amounts of negative feedback. They're constantly told they're behaving badly, disappointing adults, causing problems. By adolescence, many have internalized these messages, seeing themselves as fundamentally bad or broken. This negative self-concept fuels depression.

Shared neurobiology: DMDD and depression likely share neurobiological underpinnings including serotonin dysfunction, altered stress hormone regulation, and differences in emotion-processing brain regions.

Depression symptoms to watch for:

- Persistent sad, empty, or hopeless mood

- Loss of interest or pleasure in previously enjoyed activities

- Significant weight loss or gain, or changes in appetite

- Sleep problems (insomnia or sleeping too much)

- Psychomotor agitation or retardation

- Fatigue or loss of energy

- Feelings of worthlessness or excessive guilt

- Decreased concentration or indecisiveness

- Recurrent thoughts of death, suicidal ideation, or suicide attempts

Anxiety disorders are also common. Studies show increased rates of generalized anxiety disorder, social anxiety disorder, panic disorder, and specific phobias in adolescents who had childhood DMDD.

Why the anxiety connection:

Hyperarousal: DMDD involves chronically activated stress response systems. This physiological state closely resembles anxiety and can develop into formal anxiety disorders.

Fear of losing control: After experiencing explosive outbursts they couldn't control, many adolescents with DMDD develop intense anxiety about future explosions. They fear what they might do, worry about hurting people they love, and avoid situations that might trigger dysregulation.

Social anxiety: After years of peer rejection, bullying, or negative social experiences related to DMDD symptoms, many adolescents develop significant social anxiety. They anticipate rejection and avoid social situations.

Perfectionism: Some adolescents with DMDD develop perfectionism as an attempt to compensate for feeling out of control emotionally. This perfectionism creates performance anxiety.

Anxiety symptoms to watch for:

- Excessive worry about multiple topics (generalized anxiety)

- Intense fear of social situations or evaluation (social anxiety)

- Unexpected panic attacks (panic disorder)

- Extreme fear of specific objects or situations (specific phobias)

- Physical symptoms including rapid heartbeat, sweating, trembling, nausea

- Avoidance of situations that trigger anxiety

- Sleep disturbance related to worry

- Difficulty concentrating due to anxiety

Treatment must address both DMDD and emerging mood/anxiety symptoms. This often means:

- Medication adjustments to target depression and anxiety alongside emotional dysregulation

- Therapy approaches specifically addressing depression (behavioral activation, cognitive restructuring) and anxiety (exposure therapy, anxiety management training)

- Suicide risk assessment and safety planning when depression includes suicidal ideation

- Family therapy addressing the impact of multiple concurrent disorders

Case Example: Sophia's Transition from DMDD to Depression

Sophia had clear DMDD throughout elementary school— chronically irritable with frequent explosive tantrums. Her parents worked hard managing her symptoms, implementing accommodations at school, and ensuring she attended therapy weekly.

175

When Sophia entered seventh grade at age twelve, her parents noticed her irritability seemed different. Instead of explosive anger, Sophia seemed sad. She stopped fighting with siblings and started withdrawing to her room. She declined invitations from the few friends she had. She stopped caring about activities she'd previously enjoyed.

Sophia's therapist recognized these as depression symptoms and adjusted therapy to focus on behavioral activation—helping Sophia maintain activities even when she didn't feel motivated. The therapist taught Sophia's parents to watch for suicidal ideation given the depression severity.

By age thirteen, Sophia admitted she thought about suicide frequently. She'd made a plan involving overdose on her mother's medications. Her parents brought her to the emergency department. Sophia was hospitalized for eight days.

During hospitalization, the psychiatrist added an antidepressant to Sophia's medication regimen. The team provided intensive therapy addressing both her DMDD emotional dysregulation and her depression. They created a safety plan for home including locked medication storage, regular check-ins, and emergency procedures.

Post-hospitalization, Sophia continued struggling but with more support. Her psychiatrist monitored her closely, adjusting medications twice over the next six months. Her therapist saw her twice weekly initially, gradually reducing to weekly as Sophia stabilized. Her school implemented additional supports including daily counselor check-ins.

By age fourteen, Sophia's depression had improved significantly. She still had DMDD symptoms—irritability, low frustration tolerance—but the suicidal thoughts had resolved and her overall mood was lighter. Sophia's mother reflected: "The depression was somehow scarier than the explosions. When she was exploding, at least she was fighting. When she was depressed, she'd given up. I'm grateful we caught it before she acted on those suicidal thoughts."

Preparing for Independence

Adolescence is developmentally about separation and independence. But adolescents with DMDD often lag behind peers in maturity and self-regulation skills needed for independence. Families must balance supporting normal developmental needs for increasing autonomy with recognizing real limitations requiring continued support.

Skills needed for independence include:

Emotional self-regulation: Managing emotions without parental intervention, calming oneself after upsets, making decisions despite emotional intensity.

Executive functioning: Planning ahead, managing time, organizing tasks, following through on commitments, problem-solving independently.

Social skills: Maintaining positive relationships, resolving conflicts without aggression, reading social cues, cooperating with others.

Self-care: Maintaining personal hygiene, managing sleep schedules, eating adequately, exercising, accessing healthcare independently.

Financial management: Budgeting money, avoiding impulsive spending, saving for goals, understanding financial consequences.

Safety awareness: Recognizing dangerous situations, making safe choices, asking for help when needed, avoiding high-risk behaviors.

Assessment of readiness requires honest evaluation:

- Can your teen regulate emotions in low-stress situations without your help?

- Does your teen demonstrate any independent problem-solving ability?

- Can your teen maintain basic self-care independently (hygiene, sleep, eating)?

- Does your teen show awareness of how their behavior affects others?

- Can your teen communicate needs and feelings using words instead of only explosions?

- Does your teen take medication consistently without reminders?

- Can your teen identify when they need help and ask for it?

If you answered "no" to most questions, your teen isn't ready for full independence. That's okay. Many teens with DMDD need extended support into early adulthood.

Gradual independence works better than sudden transition:

Ages 13-15: Practice small independent tasks with support nearby. Allow teens to make low-stakes decisions (what to wear, how to organize homework). Teach money management with small allowances. Encourage independence in safe contexts (walking to nearby store, attending school events without parents).

Ages 16-17: Increase responsibility gradually. Support part-time employment if your teen can handle it. Allow social outings with peers (with check-ins). Teach basic life skills (cooking, laundry, time management). Practice driving if appropriate. Discuss post-high-school options realistically.

Ages 18+: Assess whether your teen can live independently, attend college, work full-time, or needs continued support. Many young adults with DMDD history need gap years, community college before university, part-time rather than full-time work, or continued living at home while building skills.

Legal considerations at age 18: Your child becomes a legal adult at 18, meaning:

- You no longer have automatic access to medical information or treatment decisions

- You cannot force treatment or hospitalization without legal guardianship

- Your child can sign releases allowing you continued involvement or can refuse to share information

Discuss these changes before age 18. Many young adults sign releases allowing parents continued access to medical information and treatment team communication.

Guardianship is legal arrangement where a court appoints someone to make decisions for another person who cannot make decisions independently. Some young adults with severe DMDD and functional impairment need guardianship. This is serious decision requiring legal process—consult an attorney specializing in disability law.

Supported decision-making is alternative to guardianship where your adult child maintains legal rights but agreements allow you to help with decisions. This preserves autonomy while providing support.

Case Example: The Anderson Family's Gradual Independence

Jake Anderson had severe DMDD throughout childhood and adolescence. His parents worried constantly about his future. Could Jake ever live independently? Work? Support himself?

At age sixteen, Jake's therapist helped the family develop a graduated independence plan:

Age 16: Jake got his driver's permit and practiced driving with his parents. He joined the school newspaper, giving him a structured activity. He opened a checking account and received an allowance he practiced budgeting. He started doing his own laundry and cooking one meal weekly.

Age 17: Jake got his driver's license. He worked part-time at a bookstore where his calm manager understood Jake's DMDD and provided a supportive environment. Jake managed his own money with parental oversight. He practiced independent problem-solving with parental coaching available.

Age 18: Jake graduated high school. Instead of going directly to college, his family arranged a gap year. Jake continued working at the bookstore and increased his hours. He attended community college part-time taking one class per semester. He lived at home but took on more responsibilities including paying rent, buying groceries, maintaining his car.

Age 19: Jake enrolled in community college full-time. He struggled academically and emotionally. His parents helped him access disability services at school. Jake continued living at home and working part-time. He signed releases allowing his parents access to his medical information and continued involvement in his treatment.

Age 21: Jake transferred to a four-year university after completing his associate's degree. He lived in a dorm. This was challenging—he had several major emotional crises requiring his parents to drive two hours to support him. But Jake also demonstrated growth, using coping skills and accessing campus counseling when needed.

Age 22: Jake moved into an apartment with a roommate. He worked part-time and attended school part-time. He managed his own appointments and medications with occasional check-ins from his parents. He wasn't fully independent, but he'd made enormous progress.

Jake's parents reflected that the gradual approach was necessary. If they'd pushed Jake toward typical independence timeline (leaving for college at 18, living in dorms, working full-time), he would have failed. The extended timeline allowed Jake to build skills incrementally while maintaining a safety net.

College, Work, and Relationships

Adult life involves major domains—education, employment, and relationships. Young adults with DMDD histories face challenges in all three areas but can succeed with appropriate support.

Higher education challenges:

Academic demands: College work requires sustained attention, frustration tolerance, time management, and independent learning. These executive function skills are often weak in young adults with DMDD history.

Social environment: College involves navigating complex social situations, roommate conflicts, and peer pressure without parental support. Many young adults with DMDD struggle with these social demands.

Emotional regulation: The stress of college can trigger regression in emotional regulation. Young adults who seemed stable might experience increased irritability, depression, or explosive outbursts when stressed.

Independence requirements: College requires managing daily life independently including sleep, eating, exercise, medication management, and accessing support when needed.

Strategies for success:

- Consider starting at community college rather than jumping to four-year university

- Live at home initially if possible, rather than in dorms

- Attend part-time until you're confident you can handle full-time course load

- Register with disability services office to access accommodations

- Maintain regular contact with mental health providers

- Develop support network on campus including counseling center, academic advisors, and peer connections

- Create crisis plan including who to contact and what to do if symptoms worsen

- Be willing to take medical leave if needed rather than pushing through crisis

Employment challenges:

Workplace expectations: Jobs require reliability, emotional control, ability to accept criticism, cooperation with coworkers, and handling frustration professionally.

Authority relationships: Adults with DMDD history sometimes struggle with authority figures, leading to conflict with supervisors.

Stress management: Work stress can trigger DMDD symptoms including irritability, emotional outbursts, or depression.

Finding appropriate fit: Not all job environments work equally well for people with DMDD histories. High-stress, high-criticism, or socially demanding jobs may be poor fits.

Strategies for success:

- Start with part-time work to assess your capacity

- Look for structured, predictable work environments

- Seek jobs matching your interests and strengths

- Be honest with yourself about limitations—don't take jobs you know will trigger symptoms

- Use workplace accommodations if needed (breaks for emotional regulation, modified schedules, quiet workspace)

- Maintain treatment even when working—don't skip therapy because you're busy

- Develop professional communication skills for expressing needs and managing conflict

- Have a plan for managing work stress including coping strategies and support contacts

Relationship challenges:

Emotional intimacy: Relationships require vulnerability, emotional communication, and ability to regulate emotions during conflict. These skills are often underdeveloped in young adults with DMDD history.

Conflict resolution: Relationships involve disagreements. Adults with DMDD history might default to explosive conflict styles or total avoidance.

Trust and stability: DMDD symptoms can make people unpredictable and emotionally intense. Partners might struggle with this unpredictability.

Disclosure: Young adults must decide when and how to disclose mental health history to potential partners.

Strategies for success:

- Continue individual therapy addressing relationship skills and emotional regulation

- Consider couples therapy if you're in serious relationship and having difficulties

- Develop vocabulary for communicating feelings and needs without explosions or shutdowns

- Practice conflict resolution skills before conflicts arise

- Be honest with partners about your history and current challenges

- Watch for red flags in potential partners (people who trigger your symptoms or don't respect your needs)

- Maintain friendships and family connections rather than making romantic relationship your only support

- Know that many people with DMDD histories form successful long-term relationships—your disorder doesn't doom you to loneliness

Case Example: Three Young Adults Navigate Post-High School Life

Emily—College Success: Emily had severe DMDD as a child but improved significantly by late adolescence. She started at community college living at home and working part-time. After two years, she transferred to a state university. She lived off-campus with a roommate rather than in dorms, giving her more privacy and control over her environment. She registered with disability services and received accommodations including extended test time and ability to take breaks during exams. She attended campus counseling services weekly. Emily graduated with honors and entered graduate school in social work, partly inspired by her own mental health experiences.

David—Employment Path: David struggled through high school and decided college wasn't right for him. He worked various jobs—retail, food service, warehousing. He was fired twice for losing his temper with customers or coworkers. Through vocational rehabilitation services, David found a job in IT at a small company. The work was independent, structured, and matched his skills. David thrived. He worked there five years before moving to a better position at another company. David lived with roommates, managed his own apartment, and maintained treatment. He wasn't on a traditional success path, but he supported himself and felt proud of his independence.

Rachel—Extended Support Needs: Rachel continued struggling significantly into adulthood. She tried community college but couldn't manage the academic demands alongside her ongoing depression and irritability. She worked part-time but needed frequent job changes because she couldn't maintain employment consistently. Rachel lived with her parents until age twenty-five. At that point, she moved into a supported living apartment with case management services checking on her regularly. Rachel worked part-time in a supervised employment program. She received disability benefits supplementing her income. Rachel's path looked different from her peers, but she had stability, support, and quality of life she couldn't have achieved with complete independence.

Growing up is hard for everyone. Growing up with DMDD history is harder. But with realistic assessment of readiness, gradual skill-building, appropriate support, willingness to take non-traditional paths, and continued treatment, young adults with DMDD can build meaningful adult lives. The future isn't predetermined by childhood diagnosis—it's shaped by ongoing effort, appropriate support, and building on strengths while managing limitations.

Looking Toward Adulthood With Open Eyes

Adolescence transforms DMDD in ways that often catch families off guard. The shift from external explosions to internal depression, the increased risk of anxiety and substance use, and the challenge of preparing for independence require adapting everything you thought you knew. But adolescence also brings potential for growth as developing brains mature and teens gain access to more sophisticated treatment approaches. The path through adolescence isn't smooth, but it's navigable with accurate understanding of what changes to expect, vigilance for emerging depression and anxiety, realistic assessment of independence readiness, and appropriate support for education, employment, and relationships. Your child's future isn't written yet—adolescence is where they start writing it themselves, with your guidance, support, and belief that they can build a meaningful adult life despite the challenges they've faced.

Understanding Growth and Change

- DMDD transforms across development with early adolescence bringing increased physical danger and peer conflicts, mid-adolescence showing decreased explosive frequency but increased depression and anxiety, and late adolescence/young adulthood seeing shift to major depression and anxiety disorders as primary concerns

- Depression and anxiety develop in high percentages of adolescents with childhood DMDD due to chronic stress, learned helplessness, social isolation, negative self-

186

concept, and shared neurobiology—requiring vigilant monitoring and adjusted treatment approaches

- Independence preparation requires honest assessment of readiness across emotional self-regulation, executive functioning, social skills, self-care, financial management, and safety awareness—with gradual skill-building and extended timelines often necessary

- Adult success in college, work, and relationships is possible but may require accommodations, non-traditional paths, continued treatment, realistic expectations, and willingness to accept support—success looks different for different individuals but remains achievable

Chapter 13: Hope for the Future

You've read twelve chapters about how difficult DMDD is—for children, for siblings, for marriages, for families. You might be wondering if there's any hope at all. Can children with DMDD actually get better? Will your family survive this? Is recovery possible? The answer to all three questions is yes. Not every child's trajectory looks the same. Not every family emerges unscathed. But hope exists, backed by research, emerging treatments, and real families who've walked this path before you and come out the other side.

Success Stories From Families Who've Been There

Numbers and research matter, but sometimes you need to hear real stories from real families who've lived through DMDD and found their way to better functioning.

The Morrison Family—From Crisis to Stability

When Lucas Morrison was seven, his DMDD symptoms were so severe that his family couldn't leave their house for non-essential activities. Lucas exploded multiple times daily. He'd destroyed three bedrooms, sent both parents to the emergency room with injuries, and been suspended from school fourteen times in one year.

Lucas's mother, Jennifer, described those years as "living in a war zone where we were always afraid." The family tried everything—multiple therapists, several medication trials, behavior plans that failed, school changes that didn't help. By age nine, Lucas had been hospitalized twice psychiatrically and the family was considering residential treatment.

Then Lucas's new psychiatrist tried the Matthews Protocol. Within six weeks, the family noticed changes. Explosions decreased from daily to weekly. Within three months, explosions were occurring only once or twice monthly and were less intense. Lucas's baseline irritability improved. He smiled occasionally. He participated in family activities.

By age eleven, with continued treatment including the Matthews Protocol, weekly therapy, extensive school accommodations, and parent training, Lucas was functioning at a level the family had never imagined possible. He had friends. He enjoyed activities. He still had DMDD—he remained more irritable than typical children—but the disorder no longer controlled his life or his family's life.

Jennifer shared her experience with other DMDD families: "I never thought we'd have normal family dinners, vacations, or holidays. I never thought Lucas would have friends or succeed in school. I certainly never thought I'd describe our family as 'happy.' But here we are. The journey was brutal, but we made it through. If we can get here from where we were, other families can too."

The Patterson Family—Sibling Who Survived and Thrived

Olivia Patterson's brother Ethan had severe DMDD. From ages five through fifteen, Olivia lived in constant fear of Ethan's explosions. She witnessed violence daily. She was physically hurt by Ethan multiple times. She stopped inviting friends over. She developed anxiety and depression requiring her own treatment.

Olivia's parents eventually recognized that Olivia's needs were being completely overshadowed by Ethan's crisis-level symptoms. They made conscious changes including ensuring

189

Olivia had individual therapy, scheduling weekly one-on-one time with each parent, creating safety plans protecting Olivia during Ethan's explosions, and supporting Olivia's activities even when logistics were difficult.

These changes didn't eliminate Olivia's challenges, but they prevented her from being completely lost in Ethan's disorder. Olivia graduated high school with strong grades, attended college on scholarship, and ultimately became a social worker specializing in work with families of children with behavioral disorders.

Olivia shared: "Growing up with Ethan's DMDD was traumatic. I won't minimize that. But my parents eventually realized I needed support too, and that support made all the difference. I'm not defined by my brother's disorder. I have my own life, my own identity, my own success. Siblings can survive this and build good lives."

The Kumar Family—Marriage That Survived

Raj and Priya Kumar's daughter Maya had DMDD diagnosed at age eight. By age ten, their marriage was barely holding together. They fought constantly about treatment approaches, blamed each other for Maya's symptoms, and had stopped functioning as partners.

Their couples therapist gave them an ultimatum: commit to working on the marriage or separate. They chose to commit. Over two years of couples therapy, they learned to communicate without attacking each other, developed unified parenting approaches, scheduled regular date time even when they didn't feel like it, and gradually rebuilt their connection.

Raj reflected: "DMDD nearly destroyed our marriage. We were heading toward divorce. But we realized that Maya needed us together more than separately. Learning to be partners again while managing her disorder was the hardest work we've ever done. But we're still together, and our marriage is actually stronger now than before Maya's diagnosis. We learned to face challenges as a team."

Case Example: Three More Stories of Hope

Tyler's Academic Success: Tyler had severe DMDD through elementary school. By high school, with consistent treatment including medication and therapy, his symptoms had improved significantly. Tyler graduated high school with a 3.8 GPA. He attended university on a partial academic scholarship. He graduated with a degree in engineering and started a successful career. Tyler still takes medication for depression and sees a therapist occasionally, but DMDD no longer defines his life.

Sophia's Creative Path: Sophia struggled through traditional school due to DMDD symptoms. Her family eventually homeschooled her. Sophia discovered she loved art. Her parents supported this interest, enrolling her in art classes and programs. Sophia developed significant talent. She attended art school, developed a career as a graphic designer, and found success in a field that matched her strengths. She told her mother: "DMDD made traditional paths impossible for me. But it forced me to find my own path, which ended up being better anyway."

Marcus's Peer Support Work: Marcus had severe DMDD as a child and struggled through adolescence with depression and multiple hospitalizations. By his early twenties, with consistent treatment and support, Marcus stabilized. He became passionate about helping other families facing similar challenges. Marcus volunteered with DMDD family support organizations, sharing his story and providing peer support to parents and teens. He found meaning in his difficult experiences by using them to help others.

These stories aren't universal—not every child improves this dramatically. But they're real. They happened. They prove that

DMDD doesn't have to be a life sentence of misery for children or families.

Emerging Research and Treatments

DMDD research continues growing, with new studies published regularly examining causes, treatments, and long-term outcomes. Several promising areas deserve attention.

Neuroimaging research uses brain scans to understand the neurological basis of DMDD. Studies show differences in how children with DMDD process emotions, perceive threats, and regulate responses. This research helps validate that DMDD is a real neurobiological disorder, not just bad behavior or poor parenting. It also guides development of treatments targeting specific brain circuits.

Genetic studies examine whether DMDD runs in families and what genetic factors might increase risk. Early findings suggest genetic vulnerability exists, though no single gene causes DMDD. Understanding genetics helps identify at-risk children early and might eventually lead to personalized treatment based on genetic profiles.

Treatment studies test specific interventions for DMDD rather than adapting treatments from related disorders. Several studies are examining:

- Cognitive behavioral therapy specifically adapted for DMDD
- Dialectical behavior therapy for children with severe irritability
- Parent training programs designed specifically for DMDD families

- Medication trials testing various approaches including the Matthews Protocol, stimulants, antidepressants, and mood stabilizers

- Computer-based training helping children better interpret facial expressions and social cues

Longitudinal research follows children with DMDD into adulthood, examining long-term outcomes, identifying factors that predict better or worse trajectories, and understanding how DMDD relates to adult psychiatric disorders. This research helps families understand what to expect and guides preventive interventions.

School intervention research tests approaches for supporting children with DMDD in educational settings. Studies examine which accommodations work best, how to train teachers to manage DMDD behaviors, and how to reduce school suspensions and expulsions.

Family intervention research examines programs supporting entire families affected by DMDD including parent training, sibling support programs, couples therapy approaches, and family therapy models.

Prevention research explores whether early intervention with at-risk children (those showing chronic irritability before full DMDD criteria are met) can prevent the disorder from developing fully or reduce its severity.

The Matthews Protocol research deserves specific mention. While large controlled trials haven't yet been published, multiple case series and clinical reports suggest this medication approach shows promise. Psychiatrists using the protocol report success rates above 75 percent in reducing irritability and explosive behavior. More rigorous research is needed, but preliminary results are encouraging.

New medications in development target specific neurotransmitter systems or brain circuits implicated in DMDD. While none are DMDD-specific yet, several compounds in development for other disorders might prove helpful for DMDD symptoms.

Biomarker research seeks to identify blood tests, genetic markers, or brain scan findings that could predict which treatments will work for which children, moving from trial-and-error to personalized medicine approaches.

Digital therapeutics including apps and online programs teaching emotion regulation skills, providing real-time support during crises, and helping families implement behavior management strategies are being developed and tested.

The research landscape is evolving rapidly. Treatments that don't exist today might be available within years. Understanding of DMDD's causes and optimal interventions improves constantly. This ongoing progress provides legitimate hope that future treatments will be more effective than current options.

Building Resilience in Your Child

While waiting for better treatments to emerge and while implementing current treatments, you can actively help your child develop resilience—the capacity to adapt successfully despite adversity.

Resilience isn't about avoiding difficulties or pretending everything is fine. It's about developing skills and resources that help children manage challenges more effectively and bounce back from setbacks.

Eight resilience-building strategies:

1. Develop competence: Help your child identify things they're good at. Every child has strengths, even when overall functioning is impaired. Maybe your child is good at art, video games, math, caring for animals, making people laugh, or building things. Identify these strengths and create opportunities to build on them. Competence in any area builds general confidence and resilience.

2. Teach problem-solving: Resilient people solve problems rather than being overwhelmed by them. Teach your child a problem-solving process: identify the problem, generate possible solutions, evaluate options, pick one solution to try, implement it, evaluate how it worked. Practice this process with small, low-stakes problems so your child develops the skill.

3. Build self-regulation skills: Children with DMDD struggle with regulation, but they can improve with practice. Teach specific strategies including breathing techniques, self-talk, physical strategies (exercise, cold water), and emotional awareness. Practice these skills during calm times. Praise your child when they use strategies even if the outcome isn't perfect.

4. Strengthen relationships: Resilience develops in context of supportive relationships. Help your child maintain connections with people who care about them—parents, siblings, extended family, teachers, coaches, therapists, peers. Even one solid relationship significantly protects against adversity.

5. Encourage contribution: Resilient people feel useful and needed. Give your child age-appropriate responsibilities. Let them contribute to the family through chores, caring for pets, or helping siblings. Children who contribute feel valued and develop sense of purpose.

6. Teach realistic optimism: Optimism means believing things can improve, but realistic optimism acknowledges difficulties while maintaining hope. Avoid both extreme pessimism ("Everything is terrible and always will be") and toxic positivity

("Everything is great! Just think positive!"). Instead teach: "This is hard right now, and we're working on making it better."

7. Build distress tolerance: Resilient people can tolerate discomfort without immediately needing relief. Teach your child that uncomfortable feelings won't destroy them, that distress eventually decreases, and that they can survive difficult emotions. Practice experiencing and tolerating mild discomfort (waiting before getting something they want, completing slightly frustrating tasks) to build this skill.

8. Develop identity beyond the disorder: Help your child see themselves as more than "the kid with DMDD." They're also a sister, a reader, a soccer player, a friend, a funny person, or whatever other identities they hold. The disorder is part of their life but not their entire identity.

Model resilience yourself. Your child learns more from watching how you handle difficulties than from any lecture about resilience. Let them see you:

- Experiencing frustration and handling it without falling apart
- Making mistakes and recovering
- Asking for help when you need it
- Taking care of yourself
- Maintaining hope despite challenges
- Problem-solving rather than giving up
- Finding moments of joy even during difficult periods

Case Example: The Garcia Family Builds Resilience

The Garcia family's daughter Isabella had DMDD. Her parents wanted to help Isabella develop resilience despite her challenges. They implemented several strategies:

They identified Isabella's strength in art. Isabella loved drawing. Her parents provided art supplies, enrolled Isabella in art classes, and displayed her artwork prominently. When Isabella felt frustrated or hopeless about her DMDD struggles, her parents reminded her: "You're dealing with something really hard, and you're also a talented artist. Your disorder is part of your life, but it's not all of who you are."

They practiced problem-solving. When Isabella had problems at school, her parents resisted immediately fixing things for her. They asked: "What do you think might help? What solutions can you think of?" They guided Isabella through generating ideas, evaluating options, and picking solutions to try. This process taught Isabella she could solve problems instead of being helpless.

They taught regulation strategies. Isabella's therapist taught her breathing techniques and self-talk strategies. Her parents practiced these with Isabella during calm times. They created a regulation "toolbox" Isabella could use when stressed. They praised Isabella whenever she used strategies, even if she still ended up exploding. "I noticed you tried breathing before you lost it. That's using your skills. We'll keep practicing until they work better."

They encouraged connection. Isabella struggled socially, but she had one good friend from art class. Her parents supported this friendship intensely—driving Isabella to the friend's house, inviting the friend over, helping them maintain connection even when logistics were difficult.

They gave Isabella responsibilities. Isabella was responsible for feeding the family dog, loading the dishwasher, and keeping her room clean. When Isabella completed these tasks, her parents thanked her specifically: "Thanks for feeding Max. He depends on you. You're contributing to our family." Isabella felt useful rather than just being "the problem child."

They modeled resilience. Isabella's mother told her: "I'm really frustrated right now because work was hard today. I'm going to take a walk to calm down, and then I'll be okay." This showed Isabella that adults have difficult feelings too and that there are healthy ways to manage them.

By age fourteen, Isabella demonstrated significant resilience. She still had DMDD symptoms, but she bounced back from setbacks more quickly. She used coping strategies more consistently. She believed she could handle challenges. She saw herself as someone with difficulties but also with strengths and value. The deliberate resilience-building made real differences in Isabella's functioning and outlook.

What Recovery Looks Like

Recovery from DMDD isn't a single destination or moment. It's a gradual process with ups and downs, progress and setbacks. Understanding what recovery actually looks like helps families maintain realistic expectations while still holding onto hope.

Recovery rarely means complete symptom elimination. Most children who improve significantly still have some ongoing symptoms. They might remain more irritable than typical peers. They might still have occasional explosive moments. They might need continued medication or therapy. This is recovery— not perfection, but meaningful improvement allowing substantially better quality of life.

Recovery looks different at different ages:

Childhood recovery might mean:

198

- Explosive outbursts decreasing from daily to weekly or monthly

- Outburst intensity decreasing—tantrums lasting minutes instead of hours

- More good days than bad days

- Child demonstrating ability to use coping skills sometimes

- Child maintaining friendships with one or two peers

- Child succeeding academically at grade level

- Family able to participate in normal activities (eating at restaurants, attending events, going on vacation)

- Siblings feeling safer at home

- Parents feeling less constantly stressed

Adolescent recovery might mean:

- Major reduction in explosive behavior

- Improved mood overall, though still experiencing some depression or irritability

- Successful school attendance without frequent suspensions

- Development of insight into symptoms and willingness to use treatment

- Ability to maintain part-time employment

- Some positive peer relationships

- Plans for future (college, work, training)

- Family relationships improving

Adult recovery might mean:

- Holding employment consistently
- Living independently or semi-independently
- Maintaining stable relationships
- Managing medications and appointments independently
- Continued engagement in treatment as needed
- Occasional difficult periods but overall functional life
- Sense of hope and purpose

Markers of meaningful recovery:

Functional improvement: The child can participate in age-appropriate activities (school, friendships, family life) that were previously impossible.

Reduced suffering: The child experiences more positive emotions and less constant distress. They have periods of enjoyment and peace rather than living in perpetual irritability and anger.

Better relationships: Family relationships improve. Siblings feel safer. Parents experience less constant stress. The child develops or maintains friendships.

Increased insight: The child develops awareness of their symptoms, understanding of triggers, and willingness to use strategies and treatment.

Hope for future: Both child and family believe that life can continue improving rather than feeling hopeless about permanent misery.

Recovery doesn't happen linearly. Children improve, then regress during stressful periods or developmental transitions.

They might take two steps forward and one step back repeatedly. This is normal. The overall trajectory matters more than day-to-day or week-to-week fluctuations.

Recovery requires ongoing effort. It's not like curing an infection with antibiotics where treatment ends and the problem is gone. DMDD management is more like managing diabetes— ongoing monitoring, treatment, lifestyle adjustments, and vigilance for symptom changes. But just like diabetes, DMDD can be managed successfully, allowing people to live full, meaningful lives.

Case Example: What Recovery Looked Like for the Anderson Family

The Anderson family's son Connor had severe DMDD from ages six through twelve. By age thirteen, after years of treatment including the Matthews Protocol, weekly therapy, parent training, school accommodations, and family support, Connor had improved significantly. Here's what recovery looked like for them:

Connor still had DMDD symptoms. He remained more irritable than his peers. He had lower frustration tolerance. He still exploded occasionally (about once monthly instead of multiple times daily). But the improvement was dramatic.

Connor could go to school consistently without frequent suspensions. He maintained friendships with two other boys. He participated in drama club, something unimaginable during his worst years. He earned Bs and Cs academically, matching his intellectual abilities rather than failing due to behavioral problems.

The family could do normal activities. They ate at restaurants without fearing Connor would explode. They went on vacation successfully. They attended Connor's sister's softball games without leaving early due to Connor's behavior. They had family dinners where everyone actually enjoyed each other's company.

Connor developed insight. He understood he had DMDD. He could identify when he was getting dysregulated. He used coping strategies (not always successfully, but often enough to make a difference). He stayed engaged in treatment.

Connor's sister felt safer. She no longer hid in her room constantly. She invited friends over occasionally. She reported feeling like she had a brother instead of just a threat.

Connor's parents' marriage improved. They stopped fighting constantly about Connor. They went on monthly dates. They reconnected as partners. They felt hope instead of despair.

Connor's mother reflected: "This is recovery for us. Connor isn't 'normal.' He still struggles. We still have hard days. But we went from a family in crisis where everyone was miserable to a family that functions, has good times, and believes the future can be okay. That's recovery. That's what we worked years to achieve, and it was worth every bit of effort."

Hope isn't naive optimism ignoring reality. Hope is realistic acknowledgment that while DMDD is difficult, treatment exists, improvement happens, families survive and sometimes thrive, research continues advancing, and meaningful recovery is possible. Your family's story isn't written yet. How it ends depends partly on factors outside your control—your child's neurobiological makeup, treatment responsiveness, support availability. But it also depends on factors within your control—your willingness to persist despite setbacks, your ability to access and implement appropriate treatment, your commitment to supporting your entire family, and your capacity to maintain hope even during darkest moments. Many families have walked this path before you. Many are walking it alongside you right now. Many will walk it after you. And most of them find their way to something better than where they started, even if the journey is harder than they ever imagined.

Reasons to Maintain Hope

- Real families demonstrate recovery is possible with success stories including children whose symptoms improved dramatically, siblings who survived and thrived, and marriages that withstood DMDD's strain

- Research advances continuously including neuroimaging studies, genetic research, treatment trials, longitudinal outcome studies, school interventions, family programs, and medication developments like the Matthews Protocol showing promising results

- Resilience can be actively built through developing competence in strength areas, teaching problem-solving, building self-regulation skills, strengthening relationships, encouraging contribution, teaching realistic optimism, building distress tolerance, and developing identity beyond the disorder

- Recovery is gradual process rather than single destination, looks different at different ages, includes functional improvement and reduced suffering rather than perfect symptom elimination, happens non-linearly with setbacks and progress, and requires ongoing effort producing meaningful quality-of-life improvements

Appendix A: Sample IEP Accommodations for DMDD

This appendix provides specific accommodation examples that address common DMDD challenges in educational settings. Customize these based on your individual child's needs.

Environmental Accommodations

- Preferential seating near teacher for easy monitoring and support

- Seating away from distractions (windows, doors, high-traffic areas)

- Access to alternative seating options (standing desk, wobble stool, beanbag chair)

- Designated quiet space in classroom for de-escalation

- Access to sensory room or calming area as needed

- Reduced visual clutter in immediate work area

Schedule and Routine Accommodations

- Visual schedule showing daily activities with advance notice of changes

- Five-minute, two-minute, and one-minute warnings before transitions

- Extra time for transitions between activities or locations

- Modified schedule if full school day overwhelms (shortened day, built-in break periods)

- Scheduling challenging subjects during student's optimal regulation times (typically mornings)

Assignment Accommodations

- Breaking longer assignments into smaller, manageable segments
- Extended time to complete assignments without time pressure
- Reduced homework load (fewer problems demonstrating same concept)
- Alternative demonstration of knowledge (verbal explanation, drawing, building model instead of written report)
- Use of assistive technology (computer for writing, calculator for math, audiobooks for reading)
- Chunking work with built-in breaks between sections

Testing Accommodations

- Extended time on tests and quizzes
- Testing in separate, quiet location
- Ability to take tests in multiple sessions rather than one sitting
- Access to breaks during testing
- Use of reference materials reducing frustration (formula sheets, word banks)
- Alternative test formats when appropriate

Behavioral and Social-Emotional Accommodations

- Break card allowing student to take movement or regulation breaks without asking

- Access to sensory tools during class (fidget toys, stress ball, chewy items)

- Daily check-in with counselor or trusted adult

- Social skills instruction in small group or individual setting

- Modified consequences recognizing behavior stems from disability

- Positive behavior support focusing on reinforcement rather than punishment

- Cool-down time before disciplinary discussions

Communication Accommodations

- Private feedback rather than public correction

- Choice in assignments or activities when possible

- Advance preparation for group work or presentations

- Daily communication log between teacher and parent

- Regular progress monitoring with student involvement

Crisis Intervention Accommodations

- Designated safe person student can go to when escalating

- Crisis plan specifying warning signs and intervention steps

- Designated safe space for use during escalation

- Plan for protecting other students if severe behavioral episode occurs

- Plan for student reintegration after behavioral crisis

Related Services

- Individual counseling (specify frequency: daily, weekly, etc.)

- Group social skills instruction

- Behavior intervention support from specialist

- Occupational therapy if sensory processing differences contribute to dysregulation

- Speech therapy if communication difficulties contribute to frustration

Appendix B: Crisis Plan Template

Every family with a child who has DMDD needs a written crisis plan shared with all caregivers, schools, and relevant providers. This template helps you create one.

FAMILY CRISIS PLAN FOR: [Child's Name]

Date Plan Created: _____
Date Plan Last Updated: _____

Emergency Contacts

- Parent 1: [Name, phone, backup phone]

- Parent 2: [Name, phone, backup phone]

- Emergency backup adult: [Name, phone, relationship]

- Psychiatrist: [Name, phone, emergency contact number]

- Therapist: [Name, phone, emergency contact number]

- Pediatrician: [Name, phone]

- School counselor: [Name, phone]

- Crisis hotline: 988 Suicide & Crisis Lifeline

Early Warning Signs (when these appear, implement prevention strategies)

- [Examples: heavy sighing, pencil tapping, increasingly short answers, body tension, facial expression changes, minor irritability]

Prevention Strategies (use these when early warning signs appear)

- [Examples: offer break, reduce demands, suggest regulation tool use, provide drink/snack, check if physical need exists]

Escalation Signs (indicators crisis is developing)

- [Examples: louder voice, clenched fists, pacing, verbal threats, minor physical aggression]

De-escalation Strategies (use these during escalation)

- [Examples: stop all demands, increase physical space, reduce stimulation, use minimal language, implement time-out]

Full Crisis Signs (indicators immediate safety intervention needed)

- [Examples: throwing objects at people, attempting to cause serious injury to self or others, running toward danger, complete loss of control]

Safety Procedures During Full Crisis

1. Priority is safety for everyone
2. Remove other children from area immediately
3. Secure or remove dangerous objects if possible
4. One adult stays within visual range but maintains distance
5. Call backup adult if needed
6. Call 911 if: [specify your criteria]

Post-Crisis Procedures

1. Allow time for complete regulation before discussing incident

2. Check if siblings need support

3. Debrief with child hours later (or next day) about what happened

4. Contact providers if crisis was particularly severe or represents pattern change

5. Document incident including date, time, triggers, duration, interventions used, outcome

Medical Emergency Contacts

- Nearest emergency room: [Name, address, phone]

- Psychiatric emergency services: [Phone number, location]

- Mobile crisis team: [Phone number if available in your area]

Current Medications

- [List all medications with dosages]

- Medication allergies: [List any known allergies]

What Helps During Recovery

- [Examples: quiet time alone, being held, physical activity, favorite show, comfort item]

What Makes Things Worse

- [Examples: being touched, loud talking, immediate questions, making eye contact]

Special Considerations

- [Any medical conditions affecting crisis management]

- [Any communication limitations]

- [Any physical limitations]

Updates and Review Review this plan quarterly and update as needed. Share updated plans with all relevant adults.

Signatures Parent/Guardian: _____ Date: _____

Parent/Guardian: _____ Date: _____

Appendix C: Medication Tracking Sheets

Systematic medication tracking helps you and providers identify what's working, what isn't, and what side effects are occurring.

MEDICATION TRACKING LOG

Child's Name: _____
Month/Year: _____

Current Medications

1. Medication: _____ Dose: _____ Time taken: _____ Prescriber: _____

2. Medication: _____ Dose: _____ Time taken: _____ Prescriber: _____

3. Medication: _____ Dose: _____ Time taken: _____ Prescriber: _____

Daily Tracking (Use rating scales: 1=minimal, 5=severe)

Date: _____
Medications given as prescribed? Yes / No (if no, explain): _____

Baseline irritability today (1-5): _____
Number of explosive episodes: _____
Duration of episodes: _____
Intensity of episodes (1-5): _____
Side effects noted: _____
Sleep quality (1-5): _____
Appetite (1-5): _____

Overall functioning (1-5): _____
Notes: _____

Weekly Summary

Week of: _____

Average irritability this week: _____
Total explosive episodes this week: _____
Compared to last week: Better / Same / Worse
Side effects this week: _____
Medication adherence this week: ____%
Major triggers this week: _____
What worked well this week: _____
Concerns for prescriber: _____

Medication Change Record

Date: _____
Medication changed: _____
Change made: (new medication / dose increase / dose decrease / discontinued)
Reason for change: _____
Prescriber: _____

Date change started showing effects: _____
Effects noted: _____
Side effects: _____
Overall assessment: Better / Same / Worse

Questions for Prescriber

1. _____

2. _____

3. _____

Appendix D: Sibling Support Resources

Books for Siblings

- "Siblings: You're Stuck with Each Other, So Stick Together" by James J. Crist (ages 8-13)

- "What About Me? Information for Siblings of Children with Disability or Chronic Illness" by Allan Peterkin and Irene Schumer (ages 10+)

- "The Normal One: Life with a Difficult or Damaged Sibling" by Jeanne Safer (adults/older teens)

Online Resources

- **SibTeen**: National program connecting teenage siblings of children with disabilities (www.sibteen.org)

- **Sibling Support Project**: Information, resources, and connections for siblings (www.siblingsupport.org)

- **The Sibling Support Network**: Facebook group for adult siblings

Support Groups

- **Sibshops**: In-person support groups specifically for siblings of children with disabilities (find programs at siblingsupport.org)

- **Online sibling groups**: Search "siblings of children with behavioral disorders support group" on Facebook

Apps

- **Calm**: Meditation and relaxation app for anxious siblings
- **Headspace**: Mindfulness app with programs for kids and teens
- **Mood Meter**: Helps siblings identify and label emotions

Therapy Resources

- Find sibling-specialized therapists through:
    - Psychology Today directory (filter for "sibling issues")
    - Local children's hospitals (ask about sibling support programs)
    - Your child's mental health providers (request referrals)

Respite Care

- Ask your child's providers about respite care funding
- Check with your local Department of Human Services
- Search "respite care for families of children with disabilities [your state]"

Appendix E: Provider Directory and How to Find DMDD-Specialized Care

National Organizations With Provider Directories

DMDD-Specific Organizations

- **DMDD.org**: www.dmdd.org (includes provider directory of clinicians with DMDD experience)
- **Revolutionize DMDD**: www.rdmdd.org (connects families with DMDD-experienced providers)

General Mental Health Directories

- **American Academy of Child and Adolescent Psychiatry**: www.aacap.org (find child psychiatrist tool)

- **Psychology Today**: www.psychologytoday.com (therapist finder—search "child psychologist")

- **CHADD**: www.chadd.org (professional directory for ADHD specialists who often treat DMDD)

- **National Alliance on Mental Illness**: www.nami.org (local chapters connect families with providers)

How to Search Effectively

1. Start with DMDD-specific organizations listed above

2. If no DMDD specialists available, search for providers specializing in:

   - Pediatric mood disorders

   - Childhood irritability and aggression

   - Explosive behavior in children

   - Disruptive behavior disorders

3. When calling providers, ask specifically:

   - "Do you have experience treating Disruptive Mood Dysregulation Disorder?"

   - "Are you familiar with treatment approaches for severe childhood irritability?"

   - "Do you use evidence-based treatments like CBT or DBT adapted for children?"

Finding Psychiatrists Who Use Matthews Protocol

- Contact DMDD.org and Revolutionize DMDD for provider lists

- Search provider directories at www.phillyintegrative.com and www.mindalignpsych.com

- Ask your current psychiatrist if they're willing to consult with a Matthews Protocol specialist

Insurance Considerations

- Call your insurance company for in-network provider lists

- If no in-network DMDD specialists exist, request "gap exception" allowing you to see out-of-network provider at in-network rates

- Consider telehealth options that may be in-network even if out-of-state

Academic Medical Centers Major children's hospitals often have specialized mood disorder clinics:

- Search "[your nearest major city] children's hospital psychiatry"

- Call main hospital number and ask for "child psychiatry" or "mood disorders clinic"

- Be prepared for longer wait times but higher expertise

Questions to Ask Potential Providers

- What experience do you have treating DMDD specifically?

- What treatment approaches do you use?

- Do you communicate with other providers on my child's treatment team?

- Do you provide crisis support between appointments?

- What are your beliefs about medication for DMDD?

- How do you involve parents in treatment?

Appendix F: Recommended Books, Websites, and Organizations

Books for Parents

About DMDD Specifically

- "Disruptive Mood Dysregulation Disorder: An Empowering Integrative Guide for Parents" by Scott A. Johnson

- "Clinician Guide to Disruptive Mood Dysregulation Disorder in Children and Adolescents" by Sam Goldstein (more technical but helpful)

About Explosive/Difficult Behavior

- "The Explosive Child" by Ross Greene

- "Transforming the Difficult Child" by Howard Glasser

- "Beyond Behaviors: Using Brain Science and Compassion to Understand and Solve Children's Behavioral Challenges" by Mona Delahooke

About Parent Management

- "Parent Management Training" by Alan Kazdin

- "Parenting a Child Who Has Intense Emotions: Dialectical Behavior Therapy Skills" by Pat Harvey

About Emotional Regulation

- "Self-Reg: How to Help Your Child (and You) Break the Stress Cycle" by Stuart Shanker

Books for Kids About Managing Feelings

- "What to Do When Your Temper Flares" by Dawn Huebner (ages 6-12)

- "The Anger Workbook for Teens" by Raychelle Lohmann and Julia Taylor (ages 13+)

- "Don't Let Your Emotions Run Your Life for Kids" by Jennifer Solin (ages 7-11)

Websites and Online Resources

DMDD-Specific

- www.dmdd.org - Comprehensive DMDD resource with parent forums, provider directory, research updates

- www.rdmdd.org - Revolutionize DMDD with brain-based treatment information and family stories

General Mental Health

- www.nimh.nih.gov/health/topics/disruptive-mood-dysregulation-disorder-dmdd - NIH overview of DMDD

- www.childmind.org - Child Mind Institute with excellent articles about childhood mental health

- www.aacap.org - American Academy of Child and Adolescent Psychiatry with fact sheets for families

School Support

- www.wrightslaw.com - Special education law and advocacy information

- www.chadd.org - ADHD resources including school accommodation information

- www.understood.org - Learning and attention issues with school support strategies

Crisis Resources

- 988 Suicide & Crisis Lifeline - Call or text 988

- Crisis Text Line - Text HOME to 741741

- www.nami.org/help - NAMI helpline and local resources

Organizations Offering Support

Mental Health Organizations

- **National Alliance on Mental Illness (NAMI)**: www.nami.org, 1-800-950-NAMI

  o Local chapters, family support groups, education programs

- **Mental Health America**: www.mhanational.org

  o Advocacy, education, screening tools

- **Child Mind Institute**: www.childmind.org

  o Information, resources, provider directory

Parent Support Organizations

- **Federation of Families for Children's Mental Health**: www.ffcmh.org

  o Parent-led organization supporting families of children with mental health needs

- **Parent to Parent USA**: www.p2pusa.org

  o Connects parents of children with special needs for peer support

School Advocacy Organizations

- **Council of Parent Attorneys and Advocates (COPAA)**: www.copaa.org

- o Special education advocacy and attorney referrals
- **Wrightslaw**: www.wrightslaw.com
  - o Special education law, advocacy, resources

Respite and Support Services

- **ARCH National Respite Network**: www.archrespite.org
  - o Find respite care services in your area
- **Family Voices**: www.familyvoices.org
  - o Family-led organization supporting families of children with special healthcare needs

Reference

- **American Psychiatric Association. (2013).** *Diagnostic and statistical manual of mental disorders* (5th ed.). Arlington, VA: American Psychiatric Publishing.

- **Axelson, D., Findling, R. L., Fristad, M. A., Kowatch, R. A., Youngstrom, E. A., Horwitz, S. M., ... & Birmaher, B. (2012).** Examining the proposed disruptive mood dysregulation disorder diagnosis in children in the Longitudinal Assessment of Manic Symptoms study. *Journal of Clinical Psychiatry, 73*(10), 1342–1350.

- **Baronet, A. M. (1999).** Factors associated with caregiver burden in mental illness: A critical review of the research literature. *Clinical Psychology Review, 19*(7), 819–841.

- **Bellin, M. H., Bentley, K. J., & Sawin, K. J. (2009).** Factors associated with the psychological and behavioral adjustment of siblings of youths with spinal cord injury. *Journal of Family Nursing, 15*(1), 39–61.

- **Bredewold, F., Hermus, M., & Trappenburg, M. (2018).** 'Living in the community'—the pros and cons: A systematic literature review of the impact of deinstitutionalisation on people with intellectual and psychiatric disabilities. *Journal of Social Work, 20*(1), 83–116.

- **Brotman, M. A., Schmajuk, M., Rich, B. A., Dickstein, D. P., Guyer, A. E., Costello, E. J., ... & Leibenluft, E. (2006).** Prevalence, clinical correlates, and longitudinal course of severe mood dysregulation in children. *Biological Psychiatry, 60*(9), 991–997.

- **Chen, J., Xu, Y., Zhang, J., Liu, Z., & Xu, H. (2016).** Clinical characteristics and family function of children with disruptive mood dysregulation disorder. *Shanghai Archives of Psychiatry, 28*(5), 274–281.

- **Child Mind Institute. (2025).** DMDD: Kids with extreme tantrums and irritability.

- **Cleveland Clinic. (2022).** Disruptive mood dysregulation disorder (DMDD).

- **Copeland, W. E., Angold, A., Costello, E. J., & Egger, H. (2013).** Prevalence, comorbidity, and correlates of DSM-5 proposed disruptive mood dysregulation disorder. *American Journal of Psychiatry, 170*(2), 173–179.

- **Copeland, W. E., Shanahan, L., Egger, H., Angold, A., & Costello, E. J. (2014).** Adult diagnostic and functional outcomes of DSM-5 disruptive mood dysregulation disorder. *American Journal of Psychiatry, 171*(6), 668–674.

- **DMDD.org. (2024).** Disruptive Mood Dysregulation Disorder: Education, support, research, and treatment.

- **Emerson, E., Hatton, C., Blacher, J., Llewellyn, G., & Graham, H. (2006).** Socio-economic position, household composition, health status and indicators of the well-being of mothers of children with and without intellectual disabilities. *Journal of Intellectual Disability Research, 50*(12), 862–873.

- **Fekadu, W., Mihiretu, A., Craig, T. K. J., & Fekadu, A. (2019).** Multidimensional impact of severe mental illness on family members: Systematic review. *BMJ Open, 9*(12), e032391.

- **Friedman, R. M. (1994).** Restructuring of systems to emphasize prevention and family support. *Journal of Clinical Child Psychology, 23*(Suppl), 40–47.

- **Grau, K., Plener, P. L., Hohmann, S., Fegert, J. M., Brähler, E., & Straub, J. (2018).** Prevalence rate and course of symptoms of disruptive mood dysregulation disorder (DMDD). *Zeitschrift für Kinder- und Jugendpsychiatrie und Psychotherapie, 46*(1), 29–38.

- **Greene, R. W. (2021).** *The Explosive Child* (6th ed.). New York: Harper.

- **Hannah, M. E., & Midlarsky, E. (1985).** Siblings of the handicapped: A literature review for school psychologists. *School Psychology Review, 14*(4), 510–520.

- **James, S. L., Abate, D., Abate, K. H., et al. (2018).** Global, regional, and national incidence, prevalence, and years lived with disability for 354 diseases and injuries for 195 countries and territories, 1990–2017: A systematic analysis for the Global Burden of Disease Study 2017. *The Lancet, 392*(10159), 1789–1858.

- **Kazdin, A. E. (2005).** *Parent management training: Treatment for oppositional, aggressive, and antisocial behavior in children and adolescents.* New York: Oxford University Press.

- **Kilmer, R. P., Cook, J. R., Taylor, C., Kane, S. F., & Clark, L. Y. (2008).** Siblings of children with severe emotional disturbances: Risks, resources, and adaptation. *American Journal of Orthopsychiatry, 78*(1), 1–10.

- **Lazarus, R. S., & Folkman, S. (1984).** *Stress, appraisal, and coping.* New York: Springer.

- **Leibenluft, E., Charney, D. S., Towbin, K. E., Bhangoo, R. K., & Pine, D. S. (2003).** Defining clinical phenotypes of juvenile mania. *American Journal of Psychiatry, 160*(3), 430–437.

- **Lin, J., Thompson, M. P., & Kaslow, N. J. (2009).** The mediating role of social support in the community environment–psychological distress link among low-income African American women. *Journal of Community Psychology, 37*(4), 459–470.

- **Linehan, M. M. (1993).** *Cognitive-behavioral treatment of borderline personality disorder.* New York: Guilford Press.

- **Mayes, S. D., Waxmonsky, J. D., Calhoun, S. L., & Bixler, E. O. (2016).** Disruptive mood dysregulation disorder symptoms and association with oppositional defiant and other disorders in a general population child sample. *Journal of Child and Adolescent Psychopharmacology, 26*(2), 101–106.

- **Meyers, E., DeSerisy, M., & Roy, A. K. (2017).** Disruptive mood dysregulation disorder (DMDD): An RDoC perspective. *Journal of Affective Disorders, 216,* 117–122.

- **Milevsky, A. (2016).** *Sibling relationships in childhood and adolescence: Predictors and outcomes.* New York: Columbia University Press.

- **National Institute of Mental Health. (2023).** Disruptive mood dysregulation disorder.

- **Ohaeri, J. U. (2003).** The burden of caregiving in families with a mental illness: A review of 2002. *Current Opinion in Psychiatry, 16*(4), 457–465.

- **Petalas, M. A., Hastings, R. P., Nash, S., Lloyd, T., & Dowey, A. (2009).** Emotional and behavioural adjustment in siblings of children with intellectual disability with and without autism. *Autism, 13*(5), 471–483.

- **Philadelphia Integrative Psychiatry. (2024).** The Matthews Protocol for DMDD: A comprehensive guide.

- **Platt, S. (1985).** Measuring the burden of psychiatric illness on the family: An evaluation of some rating scales. *Psychological Medicine, 15*(2), 383–393.

- **Quintero, N., & McIntyre, L. L. (2010).** Sibling adjustment and maternal well-being: An examination of families with and without a child with an autism spectrum disorder. *Focus on Autism and Other Developmental Disabilities, 25*(1), 37–46.

- **Revolutionize DMDD. (2022).** 6 things your child needs to navigate the trauma of a sibling's DMDD—from surviving to thriving.

- **Revolutionize DMDD. (2024).** Welcome educators and therapists.

- **Roy, A. K., Lopes, V., & Klein, R. G. (2014).** Disruptive mood dysregulation disorder: A new diagnostic approach to chronic irritability in youth. *American Journal of Psychiatry, 171*(9), 918–924.

- **Sharpe, D., & Rossiter, L. (2002).** Siblings of children with a chronic illness: A meta-analysis. *Journal of Pediatric Psychology, 27*(8), 699–710.

- **Stringaris, A., Cohen, P., Pine, D. S., & Leibenluft, E. (2009).** Adult outcomes of youth irritability: A 20-year prospective community-based study. *American Journal of Psychiatry, 166*(9), 1048–1054.

- **Stroul, B. A., & Friedman, R. M. (1986).** *A system of care for children and youth with severe emotional disturbances* (Rev. ed.). Washington, DC: Georgetown University Child Development Center, CASSP Technical Assistance Center.

- **Vidal-Ribas, P., Brotman, M. A., Valdivieso, I., Leibenluft, E., & Stringaris, A. (2016).** The status of irritability in psychiatry: A conceptual and quantitative review. *Journal of the American Academy of Child & Adolescent Psychiatry, 55*(7), 556–570.

- **World Health Organization. (2013).** *Mental health action plan 2013–2020.* Geneva: World Health Organization.

- **World Health Organization. (2022, June 8).** Mental disorders. *WHO Fact Sheet.*

- **Wrightslaw. (2024).** Special education law and advocacy.

- **Wyman, P. A., Cowen, E. L., Work, W. C., Hoyt-Meyers, L., Magnus, K. B., & Fagen, D. B. (1999).** Caregiving and developmental factors differentiating young at-risk urban children showing resilient versus stress-affected outcomes: A replication and extension. *Child Development, 70*(3), 645–659.

- **Yale Medicine. (2024).** Disruptive mood dysregulation disorder.

www.ingramcontent.com/pod-product-compliance
Lightning Source LLC
Chambersburg PA
CBHW071422090426
42737CB00011B/1536